To all patients and people with breasts.

To all people who care for themselves and others.

May this book empower you with

understanding to allay your fears

and create hope.

The Patient

For conversational purposes the patient in this book is referred to as "She." Men do have breast disease and cancer as well.

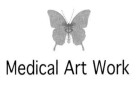

Medical Art Work
Gordon Novak, MD

gnovak67@gmail.com

Graphics and Cover
Erin Murray

Erin Murray Design

508-272-5413

Text copyright 2008, 2013, 2017, 2019 by Kerry G. Bennett

Illustrations by Gordon Novak

Graphics by Erin Murray

All rights reserved.

Published by Magnolia Publishing

No part of this publication may be reproduced, stored in a retrieval system, or transmitted in any form or by any means (electronic, mechanical, photocopying, scanning, recording or otherwise) without written permission of Kerry Bennett. For information regarding permission write to drkerrybennett@yahoo.com or check www.drkerrybennett.com for contact information.

ISBN: 978-0-578-56042-7

Printed in the U.S.A.

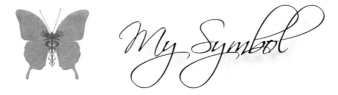

My Symbol

My symbol is on the cover of this book. It is a butterfly with a caduceus as its body. The wings of Hermes are represented by hands. I devised the symbol (with the assistance of Erin Murray) because it represents life and healing.

The caduceus is a symbol of Medicine. It also represents energy healing with the two snakes (kundalini) wrapping around the staff. These represent the ida, pingala, and sushmana, or the right, left and central energy channels. The points where these intersect make up the seven major energy points or chakras. I find it fascinating that the caduceus symbolizes Western, allopathic medicine but also Eastern, energy healing.

The butterfly is a symbol of life in literature. I was visited by a butterfly 48 hours before the birth of both of my children.

The hands replace the wings of Hermes staff in my symbol. I am a surgeon and healer and my hands are my means of healing.

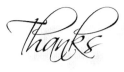

Thank you to each of my patients.

Thank you to my family especially Sam, Jack, Mom, Dad, Holly and Greg, Jr.

Thank you to Colleen Sheerin for your friendship, support and for helping me name this book.

Thank you to our wonderful team at Beth Israel Deaconess Plymouth.

Thank you to the students and residents from UMASS, Harvard, Tufts, Ross University, and MCPHS who have motivated me to stay abreast of the most current techniques and research.

Thank you to the many people who have been thanked in prior editions. This edition stands on the base you helped create.

I remain humbled and grateful.

Kerry G. Bennett, MD, MPH, FACS, CPCC

November, 2019

Thoughts on Breasts

Breasts give and receive

Breasts symbolize nurturing

Breasts change as the life cycle changes –
puberty, pregnancy, lactation, menopause –
thereby representing the universal law that
change is the only constant

Breasts symbolize female sexuality

Learning breast care equates to learning self-care

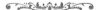

The Little Pink Book

What I Say Every Day to My Patients

4th Edition

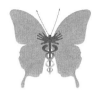

Table of Contents

Introduction		vii
I.	Breast Care Means Self-Care	1
II.	Breast Basics	2
III.	Breast Pain	3
IV.	Preventing Breast Pain and Cancer	5
V.	Detecting Breast Abnormalities	11
	A. Self-Breast Exam	11
	B. Clinical Breast Exam	14
	C. Mammography	14
	D. Ultrasound	18
	E. Magnetic Resonance Imaging (MRI)	18
VI.	Biopsies	20
VII.	What if it's Cancer?	21
	A. Mastectomy	23

B. Breast-Conserving Surgery	23
C. Breast Reconstruction	24
D. Lymph Node Sampling and Axillary Dissection	25
E. Genetic Counseling and Testing	27
F. A Final Word	31

Introduction

I am a third-generation surgeon dedicated to alleviate suffering. The Little Pink Book is one of my offerings to achieve less suffering in the world. The writing emanated from my daily surgical practice where people were so full of fear they could not remember what was said during our appointments or those with other breast health providers.

I am a surgeon who feels truly honored to practice surgery and medicine. I have immense respect for the human body. I believe the body never lies. It teaches us about common humanity (no matter what you or any patient has done, you all look pretty much the same on the inside). The body is gorgeous!! Amazing! (or as we say in Massachusetts, Wicked Awesome!) I could wax poetically about its beauty and ability. Every time I am in the operating room I am aware of the immense privilege I have to do what I do and the gifts I am receiving.

I am blessed to see many patients who are in crisis. In my breast care practice, I have patients who come in each day having recently found out (sometimes just after meeting me) that they have cancer. The word cancer fills patients with fear. Fear is no place from which to make decisions about surgery, radiation, chemotherapy, or some combination of treatments.

I help change fear to hope through honesty. I am firm, direct and kind. Through truth patient's and family's fear transforms to clarity and calm.

When we are in the Sympathetic state of flight, fight or freeze (or please) our body's normal healing mechanisms are on hold. When we drop into a Parasympathetic state our body's normal healing mechanisms flourish and care for us.

This book is my offering to each of my patients and all others with cancer or other breast diseases. It is also written for people who want to prevent breast disease.

One wonderful aspect of my work is that people rarely die of breast cancer. Through awareness, detection and better treatments (the latter apparently having the greatest impact) the death rate from breast cancer has continued to decline since 1990. But breast cancer death rates are higher than those for any other cancer other than lung cancer. So much work needs to be done. My hope is to offer prevention strategies. Women face about a 1 in 8 chance of developing breast cancer in their lifetime and the risk of its expression increases with being a woman and aging.

Part One of the book talks about the whys and whats of how breast-care equates to self-care. We then move into breast anatomy and basics as well as breast pain, that ubiquitous signal from our bodies to Pay Attention Inward Now (PAIN). I have attempted to include findings from the most evidence based medicine available at the time of publication as well as other more integrative approaches and my greater than 25 years of personal practice.

I follow with prevention strategies for all breast disease including breast cancer.

I discuss how we detect breast cancer and move into specific discussion regarding cancer.

I work extensively as a specialist in the genetics of breast cancer. And while genetics does play a role, only 15% of those who develop breast cancer in their lifetime have a family history. That means that 85% of people who get breast cancer do not have a family history. I discuss who needs genetic counseling and factors to help decide if a patient may choose genetic testing.

Part Two is a reference section where you can find the American Cancer Society recommendations for early breast cancer detection, a quick reference to treating breast pain, information on dietary supplements, and risk factors for breast cancer.

A large part of Part Two contains information on all kinds of breast problems. Because breast disease at this time is still treated based on pathology (looking at the cells under a microscope) I have based my current recommendations for benign and malignant disease on a pathology-based approach. I have added discussion on recent information about a more physiological approach to breast cancer, but at this time we do not have enough data to completely change therapies and recommendations based on how the tumor behaves. This is meant as a reference section for all patients who have breast problems.

Lastly, the book contains tables for the staging of breast cancer and additional resources my patients and I have found helpful.

I wish you the best. This book is meant to fit in your purse or be carried easily as you move about your life. I use medical terminology and define it in lay terms. Medical language is used to allow us to more specifically communicate. Like Spanish or Chinese it is another language and I try to empower you to understand medical terminology in English. I truly hope The Little Pink Book helps to alleviate any suffering you may have.

Since I wrote the first edition in 2008 much has changed in my life and in breast care. I update the book to offer the most up-to-date, evidence-based information as possible. I am honored to continue to participate in the care of so many wonderful people. Thank you.

I. Breast Care Means Self-Care

Many Eastern philosophers believe that an important cause of breast disease is over-giving or over-nurturing. In our society, women are rewarded for sacrificing themselves – for giving...and giving...and giving. But the human body is capable of giving only so much before it starts to break down. Fortunately for us, when this happens our bodies send us warning messages.

Self-care is defined by the World Health Organization (WHO) as follows: "Self care in health refers to the activities individuals, families and communities undertake with the intention of enhancing health, preventing disease, limiting illness, and restoring health. These activities are derived from knowledge and skills from the pool of both professional and lay experience. They are undertaken by lay people on their own behalf, either separately or in participative collaboration with professionals."

Some examples of self-care practices are:

Moving your body, walking in nature, stepping outside, connecting with animals, taking a deep breath and/or breathing deeply, exercising, reading, knitting, resting, meditating, mindfulness, slowing everything down, talking about your feelings, placing a hand to your heart, drinking water or tea or other nourishing drinks, saying thank you, smiling and feeling smiles in different parts of your body, taking a shower or bath, sleeping, looking at the moon, sun or stars, practicing yoga, brushing your teeth and listening to inspirational music, podcasts or books.

II. Breast Basics

The breasts are pretty simple organs, at least in medical terms. The function of breasts is to produce and expel milk and to provide sexual pleasure. They are made up of adipose (fat) cells, ligaments, lobules, ducts and nerves. The fat cells provide the bulk of what we call the breast. The ligaments hold the breast up, the lobules produce milk, the ducts carry the milk to the nipple, and the nerves make the breast sensitive to touch.

Like everything else in life, breasts change over time. The menstrual cycle, pregnancy, nursing, and gravity affect your breasts. But the biggest change in breasts comes with menopause. That's when a process called involution begins as the lobules and ducts are replaced by more and more fat. This change actually has some advantages from a medical point of view. It's the reason mammograms are much more effective after menopause than before. Women who have dense breasts – that is, less fatty – at an older age are often happy to hear they have "young breasts." The downside, though, is that their mammograms may not be as effective in diagnosing breast problems.

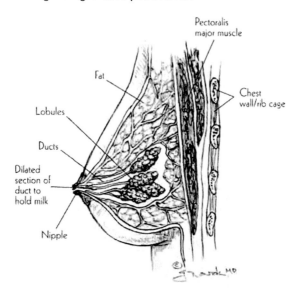

III. Breast Pain

Breast pain is a very common complaint. But breast pain is not usually an indicator of cancer. Almost every woman has pain in her breasts at one time or another, while the number of women who develop breast cancer is about 1 in 8 by age 80.

If you have pain in your breasts, they are trying to tell you something. If they could talk, they'd be saying, "Notice US! Notice our body! We must take care of ourselves." When your breasts hurt, it's your body telling you to pay attention. Use the word PAIN as a memory aid:

P	=	Pay
A	=	Attention
I	=	Inward
N	=	Now

Whenever you feel PAIN it's a signal to implement self-care techniques. After all, how much help are you going to be to your family or your employer if you're lying in a hospital bed? It's like the emergency instructions on airplanes about using oxygen masks: Put on your own mask before putting one on someone sitting next to you. You have to take care of yourself first.

The cause of breast pain is believed to be toxins deposited in the breast tissue. These come from the air we breathe, the things we eat and drink, and also from that ubiquitous offender – stress.

Breast pain can take many forms; it can be dull or sharp. It often involves intermittent tingling, or burning. Breast pain can be worsened by pressure, touch or contact with water. (Many women say taking a shower worsens breast pain at first but helps afterwards. This is because the vessels in the breast dilate in the warmth, and the increased blood flow washes toxins out of the area.) Breast pain can be so debilitating that women can't have sex or are unable to work.

Bras sometimes help with the pain because they provide support and gentle pressure, but this varies widely. Poorly fitting bras can even contribute to breast pain. Underwire bras are a common culprit because they compress breast tissue and decrease blood flow. I recommend that you avoid underwire bras for daily wear and save them for wearing on special occasions.

When your breast pain is evaluated by a health care professional an exam is done to check for any masses, swelling or skin changes in the breast. The practitioner may also recommend a mammogram or ultrasound to check for a cause. In most cases, no surgery is necessary. What is usually needed instead are changes to your lifestyle and eating habits.

As we will explore further the treatment for breast pain is lifestyle changes. These are a high fiber diet (greater then 25 grams per day), lots of water, minimizing caffeine & soda, stress management, getting good quality sleep and daily exercise. These are also the best prevention strategies to reduce your risk of presenting with cancer. Ten pounds of weight loss can be as protective as 10 years of taking Tamoxifen, an anti-estrogen drug that reduces the risk of breast cancer expression. I say this each and every day multiple times. Many don't like it and find it frustrating. Also, we can do everything "right" and still get cancer. But these lifestyle changes do have a positive impact. I know it's difficult at times but I also know it can be done from personal experience.

IV. Prevention of Breast Pain and Cancer

The best way to prevent breast problems is to make changes in your lifestyle. Exercise and healthy eating are two ways to take care of yourself and reduce the risk of breast pain or breast cancer.

Exercise lowers the risk of recurrence of pain and cancer, reportedly by 24%. Studies reveal exercise is safe and encouraged before, during and after all breast cancer treatment. It improves healing, fatigue, quality of life and overall function. Exercise may decrease hormone levels and therefore may prevent the expression of cancer. Gentle, low impact exercise such as walking four hours per week, daily yoga or tai chi, or riding a stationary or mobile bike has been found to be most beneficial.

A low-fat diet high in fruits, vegetables and fiber and low in processed food is believed to decrease cancer recurrence. How does this type of diet help? Researchers believe that such a diet lowers the insulin and glucose in your body, preventing you from gaining extra fat tissue that in turn produces more estrogen. When your estrogen levels are too high, it can increase your risk of developing breast cancer.

So when you eat, minimize your intake of processed foods. Try to eat as close to the natural product as possible. Foods high in fiber and fresh fruits and vegetables are best. Eating more fish and less meat has many health benefits. When you do eat meat, choose meat that is free of steroids and antibiotics. Try to eat five servings (where a serving equals the size of your palm) of fruits and vegetables each day. Avoid fast food places as much as possible.

Instead, eat healthy foods at home where you can eat more mindfully and connect with family.

Three major substances many people use can be especially harmful to breast health: caffeine, alcohol and cigarettes. Fiber, fluid, exercise, stress management and good sleep are the best treatments for good breast health.

Caffeine: Some authorities recommend a completely caffeine-free diet for patients with breast pain – absolutely no coffee, tea or soda. But a recent study found that caffeine may actually help prevent cancer in some people. Confusing, right? What it means is that no one really knows. It is one more reminder that medicine is more art than science and that we still have a great deal to learn.

So, regarding caffeine: What should you do? I believe the key word here is MODERATION. Try eliminating caffeine and then adding it back gradually. If your pain returns, then you may have to try to live completely caffeine-free. Or, if you are a huge caffeine addict and believe you can't live without it, try cutting back and drinking half-caffeinated and half-decaffeinated coffee. Most people are able to tolerate one to two cups of a caffeinated beverage per day (preferably NOT soda as soda as many other harmful side effects).

Alcohol: As with caffeine, when it comes to drinking alcoholic beverages, the key word again is MODERATION. Consumed in moderation, alcohol may actually be beneficial. Some studies have shown that it decreases the risk of cardiovascular disease. But what do we mean by "moderate"? The consensus among physicians is that it is safe for men to have two alcoholic drinks per day and for women to have one. That means one 2-3 ounce serving of hard alcohol, one 4-6-ounce glass of wine, or one 12-ounce beer. (And no, you cannot save up your daily allotment for the week to binge on in one night!)

The reason alcohol consumption is a problem related to breast disease is that alcohol is metabolized by the liver. If the liver is overwhelmed dealing with excessive alcohol, it cannot process estrogen properly. High alcohol intake, whether daily or via binge drinking, results in higher estrogen levels in the bloodstream. High estrogen levels are thought to be the main reason breast cancer develops. Anything that increases estrogen levels likely increases the risk of breast cancer.

Smoking: Smoking, as everyone knows, is a major health hazard. If you don't smoke now, for Heaven's sake don't start. If you do smoke, do your best to quit. Most smokers smoke out of habit, without thinking. If you smoke, try to pay attention – to be conscious of what you're doing – before and during smoking, and you will likely smoke less. Quitting smoking completely is one of the best things you can ever do for yourself and those you love.

Fiber: Humans are animals, and like other animals, we should all be eating a diet high in fiber. This means trying to get 25-30 grams of fiber every day. Unfortunately, most people, especially most Americans, do not get the needed fiber from their food alone.
Eating high fiber cereals and breads certainly helps, as well as eating fruit, dark green leafy vegetables and wheat bran. My favorite way is sprinkle ground flax seed on everything I cook. To get 25-30 grams of fiber every day, some of us need a fiber supplement. There are many on the market and they can be found at any pharmacy or grocery store. I recommend 3-4 tablets of psyllium husk or fiber tablets every day. Flax seed oil capsules (2 per day) increases both fiber and omega-3 intake. Omega-3 is found in fish oil and some plant and nut oils. Clinical trials show it may reduce cardiovascular disease, lower triglyceride levels, reduce high blood pressure and decrease the risks of breast, colon and prostate cancer.

A great fiber-boost is ground flaxseed. This can be found in the flour section of most grocery stores. Try adding it to anything you bake. I find I can add a tablespoon of ground flaxseed to almost anything – baked goods, yogurt, eggs, cereal, even salads & meats. It increases fiber without changing the flavor or texture of the food.

It's important to increase your fiber intake gradually to give your digestive system time to adjust to more fiber. The number one complaint people have about increasing the fiber in their diet is bloating and flatulence (gas). It's true that fiber will increase your gas passage. The good news is that, while the increased fiber may increase your flatulence, at least it won't smell! The increased fiber will actually decrease the odor. (And while we're on this subject, it's also worth noting that if your stool comes out like spaghetti, then you need to increase your water intake, not decrease your fiber.)

Fiber's health benefits cannot be overstated. It not only helps with breast pain, it appears also to decrease the incidence of cancer, especially of the colon and breast. It may even decrease the incidence of Alzheimer's disease.

Fluid: Our bodies are made up largely of water. We need water to survive. And by water, I mean water, not liquids in general. Drinking water rather than soda or other concoctions that are loaded with chemicals will help our bodies heal and will also prevent damage and disease. I recommend drinking water as your beverage of choice. Avoid sugary drinks and drink one glass of water for each cup of caffeinated beverage you drink.

Stress: Stress is likely the biggest obstacle to good overall and breast health. Stress causes our bodies to release hormones such as epinephrine and norepinephrine that in turn cause blood vessels to constrict. When blood flow is restricted it does not clean toxins or deposit needed nutrients as well as it should. Stress hormones also act directly to damage tissues in the body.

Learning stress management techniques and increasing physical activity greatly alleviates these problems.

What specific stress reduction techniques help? Different people find different approaches to be helpful and enjoyable. These include: exercise, meditation, yoga, mindfulness, acupuncture, massage, stretching, walking, gardening, knitting, working out, facials, drinking tea, laughing and sharing with friends. Activities that get your body moving and help quiet the mind are the most beneficial.

Women tend to over-give to others. This increases stress and may increase the risk of breast disease. I initially found it challenging to learn to sit and be quiet, to ask for and accept help but it has been worth it to treat myself more kindly and I find I am better able to give of my skills, talents and presence. Finding ways to nourish ourselves and accept support is vitally important to our health.

Exercise: We are descended from people who knew nothing of machines. Until very recently in human history, people walked, ran, hunted and plowed every day.

We have become people who drive cars and work at desks. Almost the only lifting some of us do is with our forks. I cannot overemphasize the need for exercise. It is built into us as human beings and animals. Exercise increases blood flow, helps eliminate toxins and waste, and aids in the delivery of needed nutrients and oxygen to tissue.

Walking is great, but if you can't get out for a full-fledged walk every day, try things like parking your car further from your destination so you'll have to walk a few blocks to get there. Walk around the perimeter of the grocery store and stay out of the middle aisles where all the processed food is! Take the stairs rather than the elevator. Twenty to thirty minutes of daily exercise every day is a basic goal. It's important to exercise daily. Most of us tend to overdo in spurts or force ourselves into high impact activities. This can actually hurt your body more than it helps.

If you're not able to walk, do something else. For instance, move your arms for 20 minutes. Whatever works for you is okay. The idea is to get your heart rate up just a bit for this period of time. You will be healthier, and you will have less pain not only in your breasts, but in the rest of your body as well.

One more suggestion: I advise my patients to wash off their deodorant nightly. Doing so cleans the pores which allows you to perspire, and perspiration is another process by which our bodies rid themselves of toxins. We wash our faces clean of make-up and debris every night. Doesn't it make sense to remove the substance clogging our armpit pores, too?

<u>Sleep:</u>   From college through surgical residency and young motherhood I would espouse the greatness of lack of sleep and how it didn't matter. Ah, the erroneous exuberance of youth! Study after study has shown that sleep is vital to our health. It provides the time for the body to restore and renew. Dreams help us process conundrums. Rest helps the body heal. Aiming for 8 hours of sleep, even if it is rest and not sleep, is important for bodies. Not using screens (even the phone) for 2 hours before sleep, dimming the lights, and decreasing the room temperature all immensely improve the quality of our health.

V. Detecting Breast Abnormalities

In the previous section, we looked at some of the changes women can make in their lifestyles to avoid breast problems. Now let's talk about how we can be sure the changes are working and our breasts are healthy.

These are five common tests for symptoms of breast disease:

- Self-Breast Exam (SBE)
- Breast Exam by a Clinician (CBE)
- Mammography
- Ultrasound
- Magnetic Resonance Imaging (MRI)

Let's look at each of them in a little detail.

Self-Breast Exam

The easiest, least expensive and most convenient is the Self-Breast Exam (SBE).

1. Stand in front of a mirror.
2. Lift your arms to the side and over your head.
3. Lean forward and backward.
4. Examine your skin carefully for any changes or abnormalities.

5. Get into the shower or lie in bed and feel your breasts, using soap or lotion as a lubricant.

Lift one arm. This will flatten the breast tissue and make it easier to feel.

6. Feel the right breast with the left hand and the left breast with the right. Use the pads of your three middle fingers and move your hands in a circular, up and down, or in and out motion.

(see Figures 2, 3 and 4).

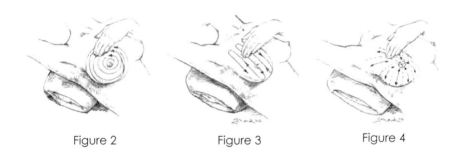

Figure 2　　　　　Figure 3　　　　　Figure 4

The actual motion is not important. It is paramount to make sure to cover the breast area from the inframammary fold (the ridge below your breast) up to the clavicle and from breast bone (sternum) to the armpit (edges of pectoralis major and latissimus dorsi/armpit). Please do not be surprised if you find that one of your breasts is larger than the other. This is normal. Almost all women have breasts of different sizes. Many vary by a whole cup size.

Get into the habit of examining yourself on a monthly basis. If you are menstruating, perform the exam right after your period when the breast tissue is softer and less tender. If you no longer menstruate, mark a particular day of the month on your calendar to remind yourself (perhaps the number of your day of birth, the first or last day of the month, or your favorite number). Be consistent.

What are you looking for when you do a self-breast exam? You are looking for a lump or area of thickening that is different from the rest of the breast tissue and stays in place for three months or more. If you find something that doesn't seem normal, it's time to call the doctor for an appointment.

Once you get into the habit of doing regular Self-Breast Exams (SBE), you'll become more comfortable with your own breast tissue. You'll find it easy to spot any changes. You are looking for something that stands out from the rest of your breast tissue, that is, a dominant or discrete mass.

There has been some controversy over the efficacy of SBE. My stance is that on a population level it does not seem to help but for an individual who finds her or his cancer through examining themselves the benefits cannot be overstated. SBE improves a person's connection to the body and does find cancers. So once per month, either on day 4 of your period (day one is the day it starts) or if you are not menstruating on a particular day of month, I encourage people to look at and feel their breasts.

Clinical Breast Exam (CBE)

All women over age 20 should have at least one breast exam each year by a medical professional – such as a pediatrician, obstetrician/gynecologist, internist, physician assistant or nurse practitioner. The typical exam begins with the patient sitting. She leans forward and backward, raising her arms to the side and overhead. Just as in the self-exam, the clinician is looking for any skin changes or obvious masses. He or she examines the patient's neck, heart, lungs, legs, arms and abdomen, checking for swollen lymph glands and any other abnormalities. The patient then lies down and extends an arm above her head to flatten the breasts and make lumps and other changes easier to feel. If the clinician finds an abnormality, then the patient is referred to a breast specialist, usually a surgeon specializing in breast care and disease. Often the patient is referred first for a mammogram, ultrasound, or both.

Mammography

Mammography is a very low energy x-ray (use of ionizing radiation) of the breasts. Some people become nervous when they hear the word x-ray. They worry about health risks from the radiation. But the radiation used in mammography is exceedingly small – so small, in fact, that any risks are far outweighed by the health risks you expose yourself to if you don't have regular mammograms.

Mammography saves lives by detecting abnormalities in the breast that are not detectable by SBE or CBE. The American Society of Breast Surgeons (ASBS) in their Breast Surgery Manual states "the primary goal of screening mammography is to diagnose breast cancers at an earlier stage and therefore potentially improve survival and decrease mortality."

Many authorities recommend that annual mammograms should begin at age 40 unless the patient has a previously discovered abnormality or is at high risk (see Table 1). If you are at high risk, see a breast specialist to determine what schedule of testing and monitoring is right for you.

Table 1. High Risk Factors For Breast Cancer

- Known carrier or family member with the breast cancer gene (BRCA 1 or 2)
- Breast cancer in yourself, mother, sibling, or child, before age 50
- Two or more close (second or third degree) relatives such as aunts or cousins with breast cancer
- Personal or family history of ovarian cancer
- Exposure to high dose radiation in childhood to age 30
- Ashkenazi or Dutch descent
- Known genetic syndrome such as Li-Fraumeni, Cowden or Bannayan-Riley-Ruvalcaba or Lynch syndrome, that increases breast cancer risk
- A lifetime risk of breast cancer scored 20-25% or greater, based on one of several accepted risk assessment tools that look at family history or other factors (such as the Tyrer-Cuzick model)
- Triple negative breast cancer (estrogen and progesterone receptor (ER/PR) negative and Her-2-neu negative)

Mammograms can be either conventional or digital. In a conventional mammogram, which is used infrequently today, the image is recorded on x-ray film.

In the digital mammogram the images are computer-generated and are reviewed by a radiologist, a physician trained to interpret mammograms, on a computer screen or monitor. The technology also allows easy storage and access to past mammograms which allow comparison of films over time. Tomography, also known as 3-D mammogram, is helpful for those with dense breasts. Digital exams produce higher quality images, improve detection, and, are most commonly used today. They also allow the use of what is called a "computerized-aided diagnosis" (CAD) system.

The CAD system is an electronic diagnosis tool that supplements the work of the radiologist. The radiologist reads the mammogram first, then sends it through the CAD process. He or she can then compare the human findings with those of the CAD and review any differences. The CAD tool has been shown to increase breast cancer detection rates by up to 10%.

Occasionally, results of the first mammogram may be inconclusive and additional imaging may be needed. The 'call back' to the radiology department may cause anxiety. However, most often, the additional imaging show that the mammogram is normal. These extra films may include views from various angles that will better highlight a suspicious area; compression views, which apply pressure to the area in question; or magnification views, which enlarge small areas so they can be looked at more closely.

What are we looking for in a mammogram? We look for calcifications, densities, skin changes and distortion. Usually these changes appear white on film. I am often asked why we look for calcifications. It has nothing to do with calcium intake.

Calcifications come from cells growing and dying and usually represent a benign process. Cancer is cells growing and dying very quickly, beyond the control of the body's immune system. The body tries to clean up the abnormal cells and clusters of calcium that are left behind. Single, large, smooth areas of calcium on a mammogram are not associated with cancer. These are called Milk of Calcium and are benign.

Your radiologist is trained to recognize the different types of calcium deposits and may suggest biopsy to be sure. Still, 80% of biopsies are benign and not cancer.

Regular mammograms are thought to decrease the death rate from breast cancer by 20-30%! If you haven't had your mammogram in the time frame recommended for you, please schedule it now.

All women should perform monthly self-breast exams and schedule exams with their healthcare providers. Mammograms for women over 40 are controversial but still recommended and definitively recommended in women over 50. The older a woman gets, the higher her chance of expressing breast cancer; so myths such as women over 70 should not get mammograms are absolutely false.

More than 95% of breast cancer cases can be detected in its early, localized state through a combination of patient self-examinations, practitioner exams and mammograms. For example, Stage 1 breast cancer has an over 99% survival rate.

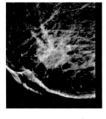

Figure 4

(figure 4) showing a classic radiograph of breast cancer revealing a speculated density

Ultrasound

If the doctor finds anything questionable in either the office exam or the mammogram, he or she will often refer the patient for an ultrasound. Ultrasound uses sound waves to make images of tissue and is very helpful in determining whether a suspicious area is cancerous. It is particularly useful with younger patients and others with dense breasts, or in cases where physical exam or mammogram are abnormal.

Ultrasound is a targeted exam. It is not a good test for initial screening but is very useful when a mammogram or exam is abnormal. It can determine if a lesion is cystic or solid, wider or taller, smooth or irregular. Solid, taller and irregular lesions are the ones that are likely to be cancerous.

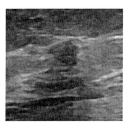

Figure 5

The black area in the center is the cancer inside breast tissue.

Magnetic Resonance Imaging (MRI)

Strange as it may sound, the MRI uses a giant magnet to examine breast tissue. The patient lies face down on a table with her arms extended over her head. Her body is supported by a wedge-shaped contraption that allows the breasts to hang free (admittedly not the most comfortable position). A non-toxic contrast fluid is injected through an IV to produce a clearer picture, and the whole table slides into a giant tube. Aside from a lot of clanking and banging from the machine, the process is painless. Unlike other MRIs, it is well tolerated even by claustrophobic patients.

MRIs are very costly and are not covered by all insurance programs. They are recommended for women with family histories of breast cancer or other factors which place them at high risk (Table 1). MRI screening is generally used only in patients known to carry a BRCA mutation, a first degree relative of a known BRCA carrier, and persons with a lifetime risk of greater than 20% of expressing breast cancer. This number is calculated using a variety of methods, most commonly online programs such as Gail, Claus, BRCA-pro, and Tyrer-Cusik models. Since the test is expensive it is important to ensure that the MRI testing meets insurance criteria as a test that is indicated in each specific patient.

Like most other human inventions, the MRI has its limitations, the major one being that it is so sensitive it often identifies areas that turn out to be harmless when they are later biopsied. (Biopsies are covered in the following section.)

MRI is selectively used for some breast cancer evaluations. It can evaluate multifocality/multicentricity (multiple locations in the breast) and is often used in the case of invasive lobular carcinoma as mammogram is not as good at evaluating lobular carcinoma compared to ductal carcinoma of the breast.

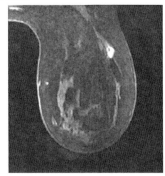

In this MRI image we see one breast. The small white area is the cancer which has taken up the gadolinium. The rest of the breast is normal.

Figure 6

VI. Biopsies

So far, we have been talking only about non-invasive (non-surgical) tests for breast abnormalities. Sometimes, though, the doctor will recommend a biopsy. In a biopsy, a piece of tissue is removed from the suspicious area so it can be examined in a laboratory.

Biopsies can be incisional which means removing only part of the suspicious area, or excisional, which means removing the entire area. When I see patients, I use the metaphor that an incisional biopsy is like taking a slice of bread while an excisional biopsy is like taking the whole loaf.

I recommend doing an initial biopsy in the least invasive way as possible. That usually means a "needle" or "core" biopsy. These can often be performed right in the doctor's office with a local anesthetic. Using a small needle, and guided by feel, ultrasound, mammogram or MRI, the surgeon removes a sample of the suspicious area and often also implants a small titanium clip to mark the spot for future reference. The entire process takes less than an hour, and the patient can drive herself home afterward. Pain or other discomfort is minimal and can be well controlled with Tylenol and ice packs. Since only a very small incision is involved, there is little scarring or other adverse cosmetic effect.

Occasionally, the location or nature of the suspicious area makes it necessary to do what is known as an "open" biopsy. This is a more involved procedure, performed in a hospital operating room or surgery center. The surgeon incises the breast with the patient under intravenous or general anesthesia and removes part or all of the suspicious mass. The patient goes home the same day and is treated with pain medication and ice packs.

VII. What If It's Cancer?

So...you've had an exam, the doctor has found a suspicious area, and it's been biopsied. What happens next?

Now comes what many patients find the most difficult task of all: waiting for the lab report. Accepting uncertainty is hard, but honestly, life is always uncertain. We just deny that fact. This is a time for radical self-care. Rest, walk, drink fluids, pray, garden.... choose activities that connect you with others, yourself, your body and nature.

Be careful with whom you share. I often tell my patient to remember, "Shields up!" because our society loves to dramatize (life is dramatic enough; we don't need to add drama to it) and catastrophize. For some reason people love to tell horror stories to those who are facing a possible cancer diagnosis. Being aware of our tendency to be velcro for the negative and teflon for the positive can help us focus on the truth. And the truth, even when it's what we don't want to hear, helps us focus on the positive. What we focus on grows.

Remember that breast cancer may be thousands of different diseases. Your truth and story is different from anyone else's. This is a time to practice living inside and from yourself to make choices instead of making choices based on how others think. A good breast care team will help you do that.

When the doctor's office calls and says your lab reports are ready, I strongly recommend you bring someone with you such as a family member or friend. You'll want to understand everything you are being told, and two sets of ears are always better than one. Taking notes can help too.

The best news, of course, is to learn that your breast abnormality is benign (non-cancerous). What that usually means is follow-up appointments for the next couple of years to ensure there are no changes. But what if it's not benign? What if it is cancer? Well, you've got a problem, but definitely not an insurmountable one. Far from it. The great majority of patients diagnosed with breast cancer go on to live normal lives. It is not a life-ending diagnosis and not time to go shopping for a cemetery plot yet. Rather, it's time to get educated about your diagnosis and your options. I suggest getting a second opinion. I want my patients to have the best care obtainable and to have complete confidence in their physician. I tell my patients "If you feel another doctor connects better with you than I do, then she or he is the one you should be seeing."

What is right for one patient will be very different from what's appropriate for another. We call this individualized treatment.

Mastectomy

More than 100 years ago, an American surgeon named William Halsted performed the first successful surgery for breast cancer. Halsted's technique was what we today refer to as a radical mastectomy. It involved removing the entire breast, the underlying chest muscles, all the underarm lymph nodes and often some additional muscle and fat beside. This remained the favored surgical treatment for breast cancer for almost 100 years and doubtlessly saved thousands of lives, but by the 1970s research was showing there were less extreme techniques that were just as effective. These newer techniques include the modified radical mastectomy and the simple mastectomy. Both involve removing the entire breast but leaving the chest muscle untouched. The difference between the two lies in whether any of the underarm lymph nodes are taken.

Nipple sparing mastectomies are becoming more accepted. Currently it is believed that if the tumor is less than 3 cm in its greatest diameter, more than 2 cm away from the nipple, and there are no axillary nodes clinically positive (that is, enlarged and suggestive of containing cancer) and the breasts of the patient are not very large or ptotic (saggy), you may be a candidate for breast tissue removal while keeping your nipple areolar complex.

Breast-conserving Surgery

Over the past 20 years, even less radical and invasive techniques have been developed. The most common form of breast cancer surgery today is known variously as breast conservation therapy

(BCT), lumpectomy, wide local excision, or partial mastectomy. These all really mean the same thing – that only part of the breast is removed: the tumor and a surrounding area of normal tissue. This type of surgery is often followed by radiation therapy to ensure that any remaining abnormal cells are eliminated. Over six major trials have proven that there is no difference between BCT with radiation versus mastectomy when we look at rates of recurrence and overall survival. Radiation is often needed after BCT to make it equivalent to mastectomy in effectiveness.

Breast Reconstruction

Just as breast cancer surgeons have succeeded over the years in developing more effective procedures, plastic surgeons have developed new techniques that make it possible for them to create a breast that comes close to matching a natural one. Many options are available such implants, expanders, and tissue flaps. The reconstruction can be done at the time of the removal, or it can be done later. It can involve implants, or it can involve procedures that create a new breast out of the patient's own muscle and fat. Many women like one of these options because it uses their own tissue and creates a "tummy tuck." The options are discussed in detail with a plastic surgeon.

Something to note, (removal of the whole breast) and partial mastectomy (formerly known as lumpectomy) both require some expertise in plastic surgery for a nice cosmetic result. Surgeons performing breast surgery are trained in these techniques to create a beautiful result. So you aren't left with a divot or hole in your breast even after partial mastectomy.

Lymph Node Sampling and Axillary Dissection

As with the radical mastectomy, surgeons initially took all the lymph nodes under the arm on the same side as the cancer, and this is called axillary dissection. It has been found that almost all breast cancer drains out of the breast into the armpit before the cancer spreads to other parts of the body.

This surgery also has gotten smaller and smaller like the breast surgeries. Lymph node sampling is done to check the lymph nodes to see if cancer has spread outside of the breast. This sampling is done to see if cancer is found in the guarding, or sentinel, lymph node and is therefore called sentinel lymph node mapping and dissection. In this procedure, a radioactive material is injected into the breast near the nipple and sometimes near the tumor. The material is taken up by the lymphatics and captured by the guarding lymph nodes of that portion of the breast. A blue dye, called isosulfan blue is also used to increase detection rates. This can cause an allergic reaction in some patients, so it is used less than the radioactive Technetium-99. The radioactivity flushes out of your body quickly.

An axillary dissection is done taking all the lymph nodes in the axilla (armpit) and the sentinel lymph node sampling takes usually 1 to 4 lymph nodes. In either surgery, great care must be taken to not injure large motor nerves to the latissimus dorsi and serratus anterior muscles as well as sensation nerves to the upper, inner aspect of the arm. The latissimus dorsi is the broadest muscle of the back and helps you extend and raise your arms up and to the side. The serratus anterior muscle is on both sides of your chest over your ribs and helps hold the scapula in place. If the nerves are cut to these areas, you may have trouble raising your arm to the side or above your head or develop a winged scapula. We do everything we can to ensure we do not injure these very important motor nerves.

A large clinical trial completed in 2011, called the Z-011 trial, decreased the number of axillary dissections we do after sentinel lymph node dissection. The study was done to see if, as with the breast portion of breast cancer surgery, less surgery can be done in axilla too. This trial has changed our practice patterns. Now if you have a T1 or T2 tumor (see Appendix VI. This means a cancer measuring less than 5 cm in diameter), are clinically lymph node negative, have pathologically proven nodal disease without greater than 3 lymph nodes involved nor extracapsular invasion, and are receiving whole breast irradiation and antiestrogen therapy, you may not need a full dissection of the axillary lymph nodes (axillary lymph node dissection (ALND)). Your doctor can help determine if ALND is needed in your case.

To check for the "guarding" or "sentinel" lymph nodes, a radioactive isotope and/or a blue dye (isosulfane or methylene blue) is injected into the breast and tumor areas. The isotope and dye are picked up by the lymph nodes that guard the area of the breast. This procedure benefits patients because it increases diagnostic accuracy and is less invasive. If the cancer has not spread to the lymph nodes, the chance that it has spread to other areas of the body (most commonly brain, bone, liver and lungs) is very minimal. Overall accuracy of the sentinel lymph node (SLN) procedure is 97%.

As we become less and less invasive with our procedures we are also finding there are some people who may not benefit from SLND, especially woman over aged 70.

Genetic Counseling and Testing

Breast cancer evokes fear in many people --- whether they have the disease or not. Fear can prompt those with breast cancer to make rash treatment decisions. Fear can cause those who don't have breast cancer to worry excessively that they will develop it in the future. Genetic counseling replaces fear with personalized information about a patient's true risk. It's another way that we can treat the whole patient --- the body and the mind --- not just the disease or dis-ease.

People with the following risk factors need genetic counseling:

- Have had breast cancer at age 50 or younger
- Have had ovarian cancer at any age
- Are male and had breast cancer at any age
- Are of Ashkenazi Jewish descent and have a personal or family history of breast, ovarian or pancreatic cancer
- Have a family history of two breast cancers in the same person or on the same side of the family
- Personally or in their family have a history of triple negative (ER/ PR negative, Her-2-neu negative) breast cancer
- Have had pancreatic cancer or other rare cancer such as aggressive prostate cancer, brain cancer, small bowel cancer, uterine cancer, melanoma or ovarian cancer

- Knows there is a BRCA gene mutation in a first degree relative (parents, siblings, children) or second degree relative (cousin, aunt, uncle)

Interestingly, breast cancer diagnosed at age 50 or younger is more important for genetic counseling and testing than the number of people in your family who have had breast cancer. To assess risk, a practitioner reviews the patient's personal and family history to determine the potential for developing cancer or for passing it on. Next, the practitioner discusses the risks, benefits, and limitations of genetic testing. Sometimes, counseling leads to the suggestion to move forward with testing and sometimes it does not. Regardless, patients ultimately make well-informed decisions.

Once results from the blood test are in, the practitioner and patient work together to establish a plan for surveillance (mammogram/SBE/CBE/MRI), surgery (of the breasts, ovaries or none), or medical intervention (Tamoxifen, Oral Contraceptives, or none). In genetic counseling, physicians and other providers look for clinically actionable genes, that is, genes that confer a higher risk of expressing cancer.

Only 15% of those who qualify for testing actually carry a gene mutation. I often describe this as an iceberg. Currently we can test for the part of the iceberg that is above the water but likely there are many genes (below the water level on the iceberg) that are genetically related to the expression of: breast, ovarian, colorectal, uterine, pancreatic, gastric, prostate cancers and melanoma. In recent years we have moved from just testing for the BRCA gene (sometimes known as the Angelina Jolie gene in popular culture) to testing for a panel of genes. We only test for genes that are clinically actionable, that is, there are guidelines on how to survey, treat and prevent the cancers known to be associated with the specific genes tested.

Many people overestimate their chances of developing a hereditary form of breast cancer. In 2019, in the United States about 268,600 new cases of invasive breast cancer are expected to be diagnosed in women and 62,930 new cases of carcinoma in situ will be found in women. About 2,670 new cases of invasive breast cancer are expected to be diagnosed in men in 2019. Approximately 40,000 women will die from the disease and death rates have been decreasing since 1989 likely due to treatment advances, earlier detection, and greater societal acceptance.

Breast cancer is a common cancer among women in the United States, second only to skin and lung cancer. The chance of a woman having invasive breast cancer sometime during her life is about 1 in 8 (about 12%). The chance of dying from breast cancer is about 1 in 36. Breast cancer death rates have been going down. Breast cancer death rates declined 40% from 1989 to 2016 among women. This is probably the result of our ability to find the cancer earlier and better treatment options. Right now, there are more than 3.1 million breast cancer survivors in the United States. The lifetime risk of breast cancer for an American woman is approximately 10-12%. Carriers of BRCA 1 have a 65% chance of expressing breast cancer in their lifetime & those who carry BRCA 2 have a 45% chance.

Genetic counseling helps people make informed health care decisions. If a patient is tested and the breast cancer gene is found, the person can take additional preventative steps. Counseling can also help people avoid unnecessary surgery or medications.

Genetic counseling and testing in the appropriate patients increases the odds of preventing breast, ovarian and other cancers. Genetic counseling and testing can create knowledge and power for you, decreasing fear and increasing hope.

A Final Word on Breast Care

Once again, taking care of your breasts means learning self-care. You are the most important person in your life. If you totally wear yourself out taking care of others, you will not have enough energy or time left to take care of yourself. When your breasts hurt, it is a signal to care for yourself. Remember, Pain = Pay Attention Inward Now.

And if you do get cancer, please know you did nothing wrong. We can do everything right and still have bad or difficult things happen. The vast majority of women diagnosed with breast cancer survive to live long, healthy, happy lives. The worst part of any type of breast disease is the anxiety that comes with it. Get help. Truly, that is the secret to a successful outcome. I suggest to get out of fear, learn the data, focus on the facts, and find trust and contentment. Those are the antidotes. Clinicians, family and friends can help you choose the treatments and life choices that are right for you. In recent years, I have begun to recommend a therapist and/or life coach to help all my patients diagnosed with cancer to help them through the acute trauma and breadth of emotions.

Whatever the future holds, live every day as it comes and enjoy it!!

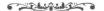

The Little Pink Book

What I Say Every Day to My Patients

4th Edition

Part Two

Reference Section

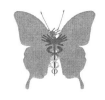

Reference Section

I. The American Cancer Society Guidelines   34

II. Treating Breast Pain and Preventing Breast Cancer   39

III. Helpful Dietary Supplements   42

IV. Risk Factors   46

V. Benign Breast Disease, High Risk Breast Disease & Cancer 48

VI. The Staging of Breast Cancer   69

VII. Additional Resources   88

I. American Cancer Society Guidelines for Early Breast Cancer Detection

Finding breast cancer early and getting state-of-the-art cancer treatment are the most important strategies to prevent deaths from breast cancer. Breast cancer that's found early, when it's small and has not spread, is easier to treat successfully. Getting regular screening tests is the most reliable way to find breast cancer early. The American Cancer Society has separate screening guidelines for women at average risk of breast cancer, and for those at higher-than-average risk for breast cancer.

What are screening tests?

The goal of screening tests for breast cancer is to find it before it causes symptoms (like a lump that can be felt). Screening refers to tests and exams used to find a disease in people who don't have any symptoms. Early detection means finding and diagnosing a disease earlier than if you'd waited for symptoms to start.

Breast cancers found during screening exams are more likely to be smaller and still confined to the breast. The size of a breast cancer and how far it has spread are some of the most important factors in predicting the prognosis (outlook) of a woman with this disease.

American Cancer Society screening recommendations for women at average breast cancer risk:

　　* Women ages 40 to 44 should have the choice to start annual breast cancer screening with mammograms (x-rays of the breast) if they wish to do so.
　　* Women ages 45 to 54 should get mammograms every year.

* Women 55 and older should switch to mammograms every 2 years, or can continue yearly screening.
* Screening should continue as long as a woman is in good health and is expected to live 10 more years or longer.
* All women should be familiar with the known benefits, limitations, and potential harm linked to breast cancer screening.
* Women should also know how their breasts normally look and feel and report any breast changes to a health care provider right away. (Self breast exam)

These guidelines are for women at average risk for breast cancer. A woman at average risk who doesn't have a personal history of breast cancer, a family history of breast cancer, a genetic mutation known to increase risk of breast cancer (such as BRCA), and has not had chest radiation therapy before the age of 30. (See below for guidelines for women at higher than average risk.)

Mammograms

Regular mammograms can help find breast cancer at an early stage, when treatment is most successful. A mammogram can find breast changes that could be cancer years before physical symptoms develop. Results from many decades of research clearly show that women who have regular mammograms are more likely to have breast cancer found early, are less likely to need aggressive treatment like surgery to remove the breast (mastectomy) and chemotherapy, and are more likely to be cured.

Mammograms are not perfect. They miss some cancers. And sometimes a woman will need more tests to find out if something found on a mammogram is or is not cancer. There's also a small possibility of being diagnosed with a cancer that never would have caused any problems had it not been found during screening.

Clinical breast exam and breast self-exam

Research has not shown a clear benefit of physical breast exams done by either a health professional or by yourself for breast cancer screening. There is very little evidence that these tests help find breast cancer early when women also get screening mammograms. Because of this, a regular clinical breast exam and breast self-exam are not recommended. Still, all women should be familiar with how their breasts normally look and feel and report any changes to a health care provider right away.

American Cancer Society screening recommendations for women at higher than average risk:

Women who are at high risk for breast cancer based on certain factors should get an MRI and a mammogram every year. This includes women who:

- Have a lifetime risk of breast cancer of about 20% to 25% or greater, according to risk assessment tools that are based mainly on family history (such as the Claus model – see below)
- Have a known BRCA1 or BRCA2 gene mutation
- Have a first-degree relative (parent, brother, sister, or child) with a BRCA1 or BRCA2 gene mutation, and have not had genetic testing themselves
- Had radiation therapy to the chest when they were between the ages of 10 and 30 years
- Have Li-Fraumeni syndrome, Cowden syndrome, or Bannayan-Riley-Ruvalcaba syndrome, or have first-degree relatives with one of these syndromes

The American Cancer Society recommends against MRI screening for women whose lifetime risk of breast cancer is less than 15%. There's not enough evidence to make a recommendation for or against yearly MRI screening for women who have a moderately

increased risk of breast cancer (a lifetime risk of 15% to 20% according to risk assessment tools that are based mainly on family history) or who may be at increased risk of breast cancer based on certain factors, such as:
- Having a personal history of breast cancer, ductal carcinoma in situ (DCIS), lobular carcinoma in situ (LCIS), atypical ductal hyperplasia (ADH), or atypical lobular hyperplasia (ALH)
- Having "extremely" or "heterogeneously" dense breasts as seen on a mammogram

If MRI is used, it should be in addition to, not instead of, a screening mammogram. This is because although an MRI is more likely to detect cancer than a mammogram, it may still miss some cancers that a mammogram would detect.

Most women at high risk should begin screening with MRI and mammograms when they are 30 and continue for as long as they are in good health. But a woman at high risk should make the decision to start with her health care providers, taking into account personal circumstances and preferences.

Tools used to assess breast cancer risk

Several risk assessment tools, with names such as the Gail model, the Claus model, and the Tyrer-Cuzick model, are available to help health professionals estimate a woman's breast cancer risk. These tools give approximate, rather than precise, estimates of breast cancer risk based on different combinations of risk factors and different data sets.

Because the different tools use different factors to estimate risk, they may give different risk estimates for the same woman. For example, the Gail model bases its risk estimates on certain personal risk factors, like current age, age at first menstrual period and history of prior breast biopsies, along with any history of breast cancer in first-degree relatives. In contrast, the Claus model estimates risk based only on family history of breast cancer in both first and second-degree relatives. These 2 models could easily give different estimates for the same person.

Risk assessment tools (like the Gail model, for example) that are not based mainly on family history are not appropriate to use with the ACS guidelines to decide if a woman should have MRI screening. The use of any of the risk assessment tools and its results should be discussed by a woman with her health care provider.

Written by

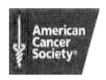

The American Cancer Society medical and editorial content team
Our team is made up of doctors and master's-prepared nurses with deep knowledge of cancer care as well as journalists, editors, and translators with extensive experience in medical writing.
Last Medical Review: June 1, 2016 Last Revised: August 18, 2016

II. Treating Breast Pain and Preventing Breast Cancer

Breast pain is an exceedingly common complaint, but a rare symptom of breast cancer. Almost every woman experiences breast pain at some time in her life, and 1 out of 8 women will get breast cancer before the age of 80.

In treating common breast pain, the first goal is to flush toxins from your body:

Diet: Low fat and high fiber. Minimize refined sugars.

Fiber: Fiber is an essential part of a healthy diet. It has been long hypothesized that dietary fiber intake may reduce the risk of breast cancer by lowering circulating estrogen concentrations. Fiber decreases cholesterol, regulates blood sugar, and prevents colon cancer. Aim for 25 grams of fiber daily (in the form of whole grains, prunes, flax seeds, wheat bran, legumes, fruits and/or vegetables). While the most beneficial way to get fiber is naturally, the use of fiber supplements is one way to help. There are a variety of supplements available; including wafers, bars and pills.

Fluid: I recommend drinking water as your beverage of choice. Avoid sugary drinks and drink one glass of water for each cup of caffeinated beverage you drink.

Exercise: Goal is 4 hours of low impact exercise per week. Some studies show that 30 minutes of walking six days a week can reduce the risk of breast cancer by 40%. Exercise is crucial to maintaining a healthy weight. Keeping a healthy weight (especially in postmenopausal women) has been shown to decrease the risk of developing breast cancer. Excess weight can cause elevated levels of estrogen, which could potentially result in the development of breast cancer. Some studies have found that the prognosis for long-term survival after treatment for breast cancer is better in women who have lower Body Mass Indexes (BMIs).

Caffeine: Eliminate or at least decrease your intake.

Nicotine: Eliminate. Another reason to give up cigarettes.

Alcohol: The risk of breast cancer increases with increased consumption. This is likely due to the effect alcohol has on the liver interfering with the liver's ability to process estrogen effectively.

Sleep: The National Sleep Foundation issued recommendations February 2, 2015 for appropriate sleep ranges by age group:

- Newborns (0-3 months): Sleep range narrowed to 14-17 hours each day (previously it was 12-18)
- Infants (4-11 months): Sleep range widened two hours to 12-15 hours (previously it was 14-15)
- Toddlers (1-2 years): Sleep range widened by one hour to 11-14 hours (previously it was 12-14)
- Preschoolers (3-5): Sleep range widened by one hour to 10-13 hours (previously it was 11-13)
- School age children (6-13): Sleep range widened by one hour to 9-11 hours (previously it was 10-11)
- Teenagers (14-17): Sleep range widened by one hour to 8-10 hours (previously it was 8.5-9.5)
- Younger adults (18-25): Sleep range is 7-9 hours (new age category)
- Adults (26-64): Sleep range did not change and remains 7-9 hours
- Older adults (65+): Sleep range is 7-8 hours (new age category)

Weight loss: Since 2013 multiples studies reveal the importance of maintaining a normal weight (or BMI less than 25). Increased weight increases the expression of breast cancer. Obesity increases the risk of cancer expression by 20 to 40%. Researchers in Boston, MA revealed data that a weight loss of 10 pounds can reduce the risk of breast cancer as much as 10 years of Tamoxifen, a powerful anti-estrogen drug. The mechanism is theorized to be that extra weight, especially around the middle of the body, is fat (adipose) tissue that produces extra (exogeneous) estrogen. The increased estrogen exposure, especially in post-menopausal women, may help cancer cells grow.

Stress management: Stress kills (isn't that stressful to read?!). It damages our organs, relationships with self and others and contributes to many diseases. Stress management can help each of us (who do you know who isn't stressed?!). Cancer or breast problems can often be a wake up call to take responsibility for limiting stress in your life.

As a long time yogi, meditation practitioner and teacher, what I currently believe is that we cannot shut off stress or our minds. We can, however, separate or dis-identify from stress and the constant stories and ideas our minds weave. We can find that inner core, our Selves, and realize we are not everything we believe or think.

Mindfulness-Based Stress Reduction (MBSR) is one clinically proven way to relieve stress. Therapy to help heal the trauma of being diagnosed with cancer can help with the emotions. I have even written another book entitled "Stress Less" because of the pervasiveness of stress and the need for its reduction in my patients (and all of us!).

Exercise also helps. Often the best way to reduce stress is to attend a class or work with a coach, therapist, body worker, healer, Shaman or other trained practitioners to help separate from the activity of the mind, connect with the body, and feel a full range of emotions.

At an American Society of Breast Surgeons (ASBrS) meeting, these recommendations were made:

- Take care of yourself emotionally and physically
- Eat healthy foods such as fruits, vegetables and those containing high fiber
- Decrease stress
- Limit alcohol
- Acupuncture can help especially with pain and fatigue
- Exercise 3-5 hours per week
- Maintain a healthy weight

III. Dietary Recommendations

A person's lifetime risk of developing breast cancer may be greatly reduced by avoiding tobacco products, maintaining a healthy weight, staying active and following a healthy diet.

** Since adding in little extras regarding spices: Turmeric is most actively absorbed with the addition of pepper. Most supplements will have pepper in the capsule but cooking may require a few twists on the pepper grinder.

Fat

Total fat intake should be limited to less than 30% of daily calories. Excess abdominal fat is thought to be physiologically active, which may increase the risk of expressing breast cancer. Try to avoid saturated fats, such as marbled meats and products containing large amounts of dairy. Fish, poultry, or beans are alternatives to red meat (beef, pork, and lamb). You can take in less than 7% of total daily calories in saturated fats (if you're following a 2,000-calorie diet that is no more than 15 grams/day). Avoid hydrogenated fats which can be found in margarine, chips, fried food, and a number of commercial baked goods.

Alcohol

Some studies show that above moderate (one or more drinks per day) consumption of alcohol is associated with increased risk of breast cancer. Alcohol may raise estrogen levels and decrease the body's ability to use folic acid, a B vitamin that has been linked to cancer prevention. Limit intake to one alcoholic drink per day for women and two drinks per day for men (one serving = 12 fluid ounces of beer, 5 fluid ounces of wine, or 1.5 fluid ounces of 80-proof distilled spirits). The recommended limit is lower for women due to their smaller body size and slower metabolism of alcohol.

Dietary Supplements

Omega-3 fats: Omega-3 fats may decrease pain and help clear toxins. They are also thought to help prevent heart disease and promote overall good health. They can be found naturally in salmon and sardines. If you take a supplement the recommendation is 1000-4000 mg per day. Omega-3 fatty acids are also found in flaxseed (1/4 cup per day). Check with your doctor if you are on Coumadin.

Vitamin E: Until the late 1990s Vitamin E was frequently recommended, but I do not recommend Vitamin E. Recent studies have shown it to increase the risk of heart disease, especially in patients with a family history of heart disease and stroke.

Evening Primrose Oil: This tried and true homeopathic remedy provides essential fatty acids and is especially helpful in cyclic breast pain. It has been around for over a century and has few, if any, side effects.

Vitamin D: Research suggests that Vitamin D3 may encourage healthy breast cell growth and make cells more resistant to toxins. Vitamin D occurs naturally from sunlight; exposure for 10-15 minutes a day usually provides an adequate dose. In the absence of sunlight, take 500-1000 IU daily. This vitamin is also found naturally in codfish, salmon, egg yolks, mushrooms and fortified milk.

Coenzyme Q-10: (also known as ubiquinone) may improve immune system functioning and resistance to heart disease. A dose of up to 100 mg per day have been suggested to be helpful in women who are approaching menopause and whose ovaries therefore are beginning to produce less estrogen (usually in the late 30s or 40s).

Calcium D-glucarate: enhances liver enzymes so the liver can better clear carcinogens. It is found in oranges, apples and lettuce. The recommended daily dose is 200 milligrams. This is equivalent to six cups of lettuce but fortunately it is also available in supplement form.

Magnesium: 400-800 mg per day may help decrease hot flashes secondary to menopause.

*Note: dietary supplements should not be used to replace the nutritional value of foods but can be used in addition to healthy eating.

Breast-healthy Foods:

Broccoli, brussel sprouts, cabbage, and other cruciferous vegetables contain diindolylmethane. This may help eliminate excess estradiol, the type of estrogen which is implicated in breast cancer. The recommended dose is ½ cup of one of these vegetables daily.

Turmeric is a spice, giving curry its yellow color. It is a naturally occurring anti-inflammatory. Add ½ teaspoon to stews and/or sauces near the end of cooking. Turmeric is also an aromatase inhibitor, which may help lower estrogen in post-menopausal women.

Green tea may decrease the incidence of breast cancer. It may also improve the survival rate in patients diagnosed with breast cancer. Green tea is rich in epigallocatechin-3 gailate (EGCG), a powerful antioxidant that can inhibit tumor growth. Adding a dash of turmeric to green tea may greatly enhance the anti-cancer benefits.

Grapefruit contains Vitamin C, an antioxidant that may help prevent the formation of cancer-causing nitrogen compounds. Grapefruit can interact with a wide variety of medicines including but not limited to cholesterol lowering, allergy, heart, hypertension, and anti-anxiety medications. Check with your doctor before taking any supplements or changing your diet.

Pomegranates are full of ellagic acid, a dietary-derived polyphenol. Ellagic acid may prevent cell growth of cancer and deactivate cancer causing compounds.

Shitake and maitake mushrooms are other foods that may help prevent cancer by boosting the body's immune system, especially natural killer cells.

Disclaimer: This information is not to be used as a substitute for any medical advice, diagnosis, or treatment of any health condition or problem. Any questions in regard to your own health should be addressed by your physician or other healthcare provider. Information related to health changes frequently. Therefore, information noted here may be outdated, incomplete or incorrect. It is important to keep in mind that studies regarding breast health may be conflicting. You are advised to consult with your physician or another professional healthcare provider prior to making any decisions, or taking actions related to any healthcare problem or issue you might have at any time.

Thank you Laurelle Tetreault for your research and writing of this section.

IV. Risk Factors

The major risk factor for breast cancer is increased estrogen exposure. Increased estrogen exposure comes in a variety of forms. Many of these forms we cannot change such as when we first get our periods (called menarche) or when we enter menopause. But we can lower some forms of increased estrogen exposure by maintaining a healthy weight and limiting alcohol consumption.

Other Risk Factors for Breast Cancer:

*Demographic Factors:
- Age greater than 30
- Female gender

*Greatly increased risk:
- Known carrier of BRCA 1 or 2 or family member of known carrier
- Strong family history (2+ relatives) with bilateral or premenopausal breast cancer
- Previously diagnosed ADH, ALH, DCIS, LCIS or breast cancer

*Moderately increased risk:
- Family history - one or more relatives with breast cancer, not bilateral or premenopausal
- Menstrual history – menarche (start of menstruation) before 12 years old and/or menopause after 55 years old
- Parity – nulliparity (never gave birth) or had first live full-term birth after age 30
- Radiation – exposure to low dose ionizing radiation in childhood or adolescence, especially in the chest area
- Other cancers in yourself or family such as colon, ovarian, endometrial, pancreatic or brain cancer (including meningioma)
- A high fat or high calorie diet
- Obesity especially around abdomen which increases estrogenization
- Hormone Replacement Therapy (HRT)

You cannot change your age, family history, when you began or stopped having periods, previous cancer diagnoses or genetic makeup. You can change your diet and lifestyle habits. Do not take HRT beyond age 50 for longer than 2 years. If you have ever been diagnosed with cancer or a precancerous lesion such as LCIS, ALH or ADH do not take oral HRT. Vaginal application of estrogen may be okay but is not well researched.

V. <u>Benign Breast Disease, High Risk Breast Disease & Breast Cancer</u>

Breast disease is categorized by how it looks on pathology slides. We remove the tissue and look at it under a microscope. This lets us know what is happening in the breast. Clinicians then tailor treatments based on the tissue diagnosis and current research.

In talking about breast disease, I use the medical terms and try to define them so you become more fluent in medical terminology. It is a different language, like Chinese, Spanish, or English, with the purpose of clearly and specifically communicating. I believe it is important for patients to begin to learn medical language to ensure better diagnosis and treatment. Herein, you will find the common pathologic diagnoses with their descriptions, treatments and my guidance. I have categorized them into three main topics: benign breast disease, high risk breast disease and breast cancer.

BENIGN BREAST DISEASE

I. Fibrocystic Changes
II. Breast Cysts
III. Fibroadenoma
IV. Papilloma
V. Sclerosing Lesions
VI. Gynecomastia
VII. Phylloides Tumors
VIII. Pseudoangiomatous Stromal Hyperplasia (PASH)

I. FIBROCYSTIC CHANGES

Fibrocystic changes have main causes and findings. In medical language, we say fibrocystic changes contain a spectrum of clinical and histological findings. They include breasts that have cyst formation, breast nodularity, tissue growth and proliferation, and duct and lobule cell growth (epithelial hyperplasia).

Breasts may feel bumpy or nodular. More than half of women experience these changes during their lifetime. Bumpy or nodular breasts are not considered a disease, but a change many women have. Breast tissue can grow in response to hormones, stress and toxins. Pathologically we can see macrocysts (big cysts), microcysts (small cysts), stromal fibrosis (increased hard noncancerous tissue), epithelial metaplasia (changes in the cells), and hyperplasia (increased growth of the cells).

The mainstay of treatment is self-care. A high fiber diet, drinking water, moving your body and getting enough sleep can alleviate the discomfort associated with these changes.

II. BREAST CYSTS

Cysts are common and occur most frequently in women ages 35-50. Breast cysts often occur at times of great hormonal change such as puberty, pregnancy and menopause. From an emotional standpoint, breast cysts, lumps and soreness are thought to result from a lack of self-nourishment and putting everyone else first.

Pathologically, cysts are simple or complex. Imagine a circle. A simple cyst is just one circle. A complex cyst is a collection of circles of various sizes all bunched and connected together. Another way to imagine this is to imagine one office (simple cyst) within a whole floor office space (complex cyst).

We can observe, drain or remove breast cysts. First, the clinician examines the patient. Ultrasound better characterizes cysts. On an ultrasound image a cyst will look black on the inside with a white outside that becomes very white on one side. The sound waves from the ultrasound transmit through the fluid, making it look whiter on the deepest side. Small cysts are often watched and treated using the recommendations in Parts II and III (treating breast pain and possible helpful dietary supplements) of this book's reference section. Basic treatment includes a high fiber and low fat diet, daily movement, increased water intake, good sleep and stress management techniques. To be effective, these approaches need to be practiced consistently and over time.

Larger cysts can be aspirated (drained) with or without the help of ultrasound guidance. If the fluid within the cyst is clear, green or yellow it is discarded and the patient may return in 3-6 months for a follow up exam. If the fluid is bloody, it is sent for cytology (a laboratory analysis) and follow up occurs sooner. I typically will drain non-bloody cysts twice. If they recur more than twice, have symptoms such as pain or growth, or the patient has immense anxiety, I often proceed with cyst removal (also referred to as an excision) during a same day surgery.

III. FIBROADENOMA

A fibroadenoma is a benign breast mass containing stromal and epithelial elements. In non-medical terminology, it is a non-cancerous mass made up of breast tissue arranged in an abnormal fashion. Fibroadenomas are the second most common solid tumor of the breast (second to breast cancer). They are most commonly seen in women less than 30 years old, especially those in their teenage years.

Hamartomas and adenomas are similar to fibroadenomas. They are benign masses containing variable amounts of epithelial and stromal tissue. They are indistinguishable from fibroadenomas on work up but are found at pathology to be different. Traditionally, these masses were left in the breast. Currently, we recommend excision if the mass is greater than 1.5 cm in width, causes symptoms, is newly appearing in women older than 35, causes patient anxiety, or to establish definitive pathologic diagnosis. These masses may decrease the risk of pre-invasive cancer. However, in general they are thought not to have an association with cancer.

IV. PAPILLOMA

Papilloma's are true polyps of the breast ducts. They are often located under the areola (nipple complex) and cause a bloody nipple discharge. The treatment is total excision through a circumareolar (around the nipple areolar complex) incision. Papillomatosis is not a true papilloma and is categorized as a type of fibrocystic change. These lesions do not directly lead to cancer. Any risk of cancer is associated with the degree of atypical epithelial cells, abnormal ductal or lobular cells seen at pathology.

V. SCLEROSING LESIONS

1. Sclerosing Adenosis

Sclerosing means scarring and adenosis means an increased number of small terminal ductules or acini. This means that the ducts at their ends become obliterated. The tissue around the scarring ducts increases. Theoretically, this can stimulate the growth of abnormal cells, but this process has not been found to increase the risk of cancer in individual patients. Often calcium is depositing in the area reflecting the death of the cells in the area. The calcium deposits make it easier to identify on mammogram.

2. Radical Scar

Radical scar is a benign group of related abnormalities known as complex sclerosing adenosis. It can mimic cancer on a mammogram or during physical exam. Pathologically, scar or sclerosis is seen centrally with surrounding small cysts, epithelial hyperplasia (increased growth of cells) and adenosis (see above). The presentation can be confusing and concerning, but the lesion itself is benign and not cancer.

3. Fat Necrosis

Fat necrosis comes from trauma to the breast. Often women present with a breast mass after being in a crowded, public place such as Disney World or after taking care of a child or animal that jumped on her chest. The mass feels hard and does not move. Sometimes it hurts, at other times it does not. Women usually have no memory of any trauma or hit. On presentation, fat necrosis can mimic cancer because it feels hard, immobile and irregular. On mammogram, a density, calcification and/or skin distortion, all findings consistent with cancer, can be seen. This is not an epithelial (ductal or lobular) lesion but a reaction of the fat to trauma and pressure. There is no malignant potential.

VI. GYNECOMASTIA

Gynecomastia occurs in men when the glandular breast tissue proliferates and grows. It occurs most commonly in newborns, adolescents and the elderly. If it occurs only on one side it should be evaluated by a breast clinician and perhaps biopsied, especially if the breast tissue is hard and painless.

Enlarged breasts in men can occur from genetic syndromes, hormones (from excess fat, tumors or injected), liver or kidney problems, hyperthyroidism and many medications. Obesity can cause the breasts to appear enlarged but that is not true gynecomastia because in that case fat is in the breast area but it is not a true proliferation of the breast glandular tissue.

On exam, gynecomastia will feel rubbery and like a disc right below the nipple. Tests that may help are mammogram and/or ultrasound as well as core biopsy of the area. Treatments include Tamoxifen (used rarely), medication change or discontinuation, weight loss and dietary changes, treating the primary medical problem and sometimes surgery to remove the area, especially if longstanding.

VII. PHYLLOIDES TUMORS

Phylloides means leaf and these tumors look like a leaf when seen under the microscope. They are very rare (less than 1% of breast lesions) and are almost always benign. They present in women and have a high rate of recurrence. They can look like a fibroadenoma on ultrasound and physical exam but tend to be large (>4cm) or grow quickly. Treatment is removal with sometimes with at least 1 cm margins to help decrease recurrence.

VIII. PSEUDOANGIOMATOUS STROMAL HYPERPLASIA (PASH)

Pseudoangiomatous stromal hyperplasia (PASH) is a non-cancerous growth of breast tissue and is often found on core biopsy of mammographically detected lesions. It does not increase the risk of breast cancer but is often excised via an open surgical approach to ensure it is not cancer.

HIGH RISK BREAST DISEASE

I. Nipple Discharge
II. Florid Ductal Hyperplasia
III. Atypical Lobular Hyperplasia (ALH)
IV. Atypical Ductal Hyperplasia (ADH)
V. Lobular Carcinoma In Situ (LCIS)
VI. Ductal Carcinoma In Situ (DCIS)
VII. Breast Cancer

I. NIPPLE DISCHARGE

The choice of whether to put nipple discharge in the benign or high risk disease category can be difficult. Nipple discharge comes in many colors including red, clear, white, yellow and green. The most common type of nipple discharge is milk from nursing mothers. Red or bloody nipple discharge is most commonly associated with a benign lesion called intraductal papilloma which is treated with surgery. Sometimes it is associated with cancer and, therefore, always needs to be evaluated. Non-bloody nipple discharge is considered benign. It most commonly occurs with nipple stimulation. The stimulation is often from sexual or self-manipulation. Other times or concurrently the discharge occurs from ill-fitting bras or clothes rubbing the nipple areolar complex.

Persistent nipple discharge, especially in those who have not nursed in over a year, needs to be evaluated with hormonal studies. Most commonly, the prolactin level and thyroid hormones are checked. Abnormal hormonal levels are rare and if they cause the nipple discharge the etiology (cause) needs to be treated.

Cancer is associated with nipple discharge about 5-15% of the time. We worry most if the discharge is unilateral, spontaneous, serous or bloody. First tests performed are a physical exam, mammogram and ultrasound. Cytology (laboratory analysis of cells) has not been found to be very helpful in the diagnosis. Other tests that nowadays are rarely used are ductography (injecting dye into the duct during an x-ray), ductoscopy (used mainly be centers investigating whether looking inside the duct with a small camera will help) and wire probe and/or dye excision (using a probe or dye to remove the involved duct).

II. FLORID DUCTAL HYPERPLASIA

Florid ductal hyperplasia literally means a lot of increased growth of the ducts. The major anatomical tissues of the breast are adipose (fat) cells, lobules (which produce the milk), ducts (which carry the milk from the lobules out through the nipple), and ligaments (which are affected by gravity as we age and lose their strength). In florid ductal hyperplasia, the ductal cells begin to grow in abundance without any atypia (abnormal looking cells). If diagnosed by a core biopsy an open biopsy is recommended to ensure accurate diagnosis. Patients who have been found to have this condition may be followed with SBE monthly, CBE 1-2 times per year and an annual mammogram unless their personal or family history includes them in a high-risk category requiring additional surveillance.

Premalignant and In Situ Disease of the Breast

Premalignant disease means abnormalities of the breast that indicate a high risk of developing breast cancer. Table 2 lists the majority of these diseases and the amount of risk they confer. Of note, lobular and ductal disease behave very differently. In brief, lobular disease in situ is considered to be a marker of developing cancer in the future and not cancer in and of itself. Ductal disease in situ is thought to progress into invasive disease and is considered to be a type of breast cancer. Therefore, we want "negative margins" with ductal disease. That means no abnormal cells at the edge of the specimen. Exactly how far from the edge is controversial. Even 1 mm or less is now considered acceptable as a "negative margin."

Table 2.

Breast Condition	Risk
Non-proliferative lesions	No increased risk
Intraductal papilloma	No increased risk
Sclerosing adenosis	No increased risk
Florid ductal hyperplasia	1.5 to 2-fold increase
ALH	4-fold increase
ADH	4-fold increase
LCIS	10-fold increase
DCIS	10-fold increase

III. ATYPICAL LOBULAR HYPERPLASIA (ALH)

Atypical lobular hyperplasia (ALH) means increased growth of the lobular cells (enlargement of the terminal duct lobular unit) and some of the cells look abnormal. This is determined by the pathologist. This diagnosis fulfills some, but not all, of the criteria of lobular carcinoma in situ (LCIS) (see below). The risk of developing a subsequent invasive cancer (usually of ductal type) is four times higher than the risk of women who do not carry the diagnosis of ALH. It most commonly occurs in women who are pre- or peri-menopausal (before or around menopause). If a woman has a family history of breast cancer and ALH, her risk is 8 times that of the general population. ALH is thought to be a marker of disease. That is, if left alone it will likely not progress into a cancer. Rather, people with ALH have a higher chance of getting breast cancer in any of the breast tissue. If cancer develops the pathology type is not necessarily lobular. The cancers that occur in patients with ALH follow that of the general population: 80% invasive ductal and 20% invasive lobular. Open surgical excision is individualized f ALH is found on core biopsy.

IV. ATYPICAL DUCTAL HYPERPLASIA (ADH)

Atypical ductal hyperplasia (ADH) means increased growth of the ductal cells (proliferation of the terminal duct unit) and some of the cells look abnormal. Again, this is determined by the pathologist. These cells do not meet the criteria for ductal carcinoma in situ (DCIS) (see below). The natural history suggests an intermediate increased risk for the development of breast cancer (four-fold risk).

Ten percent of women with ADH will develop invasive carcinoma over a 10-15-year period after biopsy. These patients need to see a Medical Oncologist for preventive strategies such as anti-hormone therapy. In contrast to ALH, it is thought that if ADH is left alone, it could progress into DCIS and then invasive ductal cancer. Therefore, it is excised more frequently than ALH if found on core biopsy.

V. & VI. LOBULAR CARCINOMA IN SITU AND DUCTAL CARCINOMA IN SITU (LCIS & DCIS)

The normal duct and lobule each have one cell layer. (see Figure 5). Think of a duct as a tube where the cells represent the lining of the tube. When cells begin to grow outside of the body's normal control mechanisms, the cell layer becomes thicker, like a tube getting gunk in it. This is "in situ" disease (see Figure 6). When the abnormal cells (the gunk on the inside of the tube) keep growing, they start growing outside the tube and into the tissue surrounding the tube. That is invasive cancer. (see Figure 7).

Figure 5

Figure 6

Figure 7

V. LCIS

Lobular carcinoma in situ (LCIS) is thought to be a marker of disease. If it is found, that person has a 10-fold increased chance of expressing cancer in either breast. Even clinicians find this confusing. As with ALH, negative margins are not thought to be necessary, although if found on core biopsy, open biopsy should still be performed for diagnostic accuracy. Finding these types of cells in a breast immediately qualifies this person as high risk for the development of breast cancer. The high-risk recommendations currently recommend SBE monthly, CBE two times per year, annual mammogram and annual MRI, spaced six months apart. These patients are also referred to a medical oncologist for follow-up and possible drug therapy for prevention, such as Tamoxifen.

VI. DCIS

Ductal Carcinoma in situ (DCIS) often is found on mammogram as calcifications. All DCIS must be removed surgically to prevent early recurrence. It is thought that if DCIS, in contrast to LCIS, is left behind, it may progress into invasive breast cancer. Sometimes DCIS is treated with surgical excision alone. This usually requires a margin of 2mm or more and is done most commonly in patients who have more complex medical problems and greater age.

Most commonly, DCIS is treated with removal of the abnormal area with negative margins and radiation therapy. The radiation therapy usually lasts for five days per week for three to six weeks. The most common side effects of radiation treatment are irritation of the skin and fatigue. Full breast radiation has been the standard care for prevention although partial breast radiation is currently being investigated and used in some centers. Frequently, these patients also receive a preventive medication such as Tamoxifen or an aromatase inhibitor prescribed by a medical oncologist. DCIS is considered to be an early, non-invading form of breast cancer and is often called Stage Zero breast cancer.

VII. BREAST CANCER

Breast cancer is malignant abnormal cell growth in the breast. It is the second most common type of cancer in the United States but the most common cancer globally in women. Its incidence increases after age 40. The risk factors for getting breast cancer are: being a woman, increasing age, exposure to estrogen and a personal or family history of breast cancer.

Breast cancer is usually of ductal type. There are two main types of cells that become cancerous in the breast: the ducts and the lobules. The lobule is where milk is produced and the ducts carry the milk from the lobules out through the nipple. Invasive ductal carcinoma represents 70-80% of all cases of breast cancer. A breast cancer is deemed invasive when it invades outside of the duct or lobule lining, which is called the basement membrane (see Figure 8 on page 58).

Cancer may be associated with calcifications, a density or a mass on physical exam, mammogram or ultrasound. There are things we feel and things we see. Only a subset of breast problems is felt and seen (see Figure 8). Calcifications appear as white dots on mammogram. They come from cells growing and dying faster than normal. Your body's immune system cleans away abnormal cells. Cancer occurs when your body's immune system can't keep up. As your body is trying to eliminate cancer, it leaves behind waste. The waste can sometimes be seen as calcifications on mammogram. Not all calcifications are cancer.

Genetic counseling and testing, if chosen, should be carried out on all patients 50 years old with a diagnosis of DCIS or invasive cancer.

Figure 8

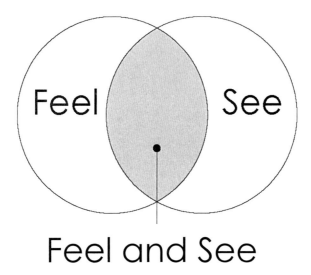

Treatment based on pathology

Invasive ductal and lobular cancer are both treated the same way. The diagnosis is made by the pathologist who looks at the tissue for specific characteristics. The pathologist will test the tissue to see if it expresses estrogen or progesterone receptors. If the tissue does produce these receptors, a medical oncologist may be able to prescribe anti-hormone therapies, such as Tamoxifen, or an aromatase inhibitor, such as Femara, to help prevent the cancer from growing or coming back.

The pathologist will also check the tissue for Her-2-neu. Her-2-neu is a genetic marker of breast cancer termed an oncogene (cancer gene). Normal cells have two copies of the Her-2-neu gene and low levels of the Her-2 protein. Some breast cancers have more copies of the gene and, therefore, more protein. Tumors that have more Her-2-neu tend to be more aggressive. It is classified as 1+, 2+, or 3+. 1+ means there is not much Her-2-neu while 3+ means there is more Her-2-neu. Tumors that test as 2+ will be retested through an assay called "FISH" analysis to determine if they fall into category 1+ or 3+. The tumors that are Her-2-neu positive can be treated with a special form of chemotherapy called Herceptin.

Types of breast cancer include:
- Ductal carcinoma in situ (DCIS)
- Paget's disease (a skin lesion that will not heal of the nipple areolar complex that appears red/white and scaly that can itch, bleed, or hurt)

- Invasive cancer (ductal = 75%, lobular = 10%, ductal and lobular = 10%, colloid 1-2%, tubular 1-2% [colloid and tubular have more favorable prognosis])

Figure 9

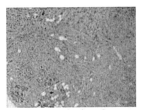

Invasive Lobular Cancer

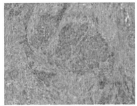

Invasive Ductal Cancer

- Inflammatory breast cancer (1-6%) (The breast may become large, swollen, red or look like the skin of an orange with rapid onset of symptoms and may be confused with infection of the breast.)

Most breast cancer does not cause pain and is found on screening mammogram. You can do everything right in life and still get cancer. Mammograms will find cancers when they are small. Sometimes cancers are felt (palpable) or cause the nipple to be retracted or the skin to be dimpled.

<u>Surgery, Radiation & Chemotherapy</u>

The mainstay of breast cancer treatment is surgery. Depending on the size of the tumor and of the breast, the patient will have to decide if she is going to have a mastectomy (removal of the whole breast) or a partial mastectomy (sometimes called a lumpectomy). If she chooses a partial, (which is full removal of the cancer with negative margins) she will undergo radiation therapy for six weeks or undergo a newer, less available therapy called partial breast irradiation for five days. Full breast radiation is most commonly done today. This usually starts about one month after surgery. If the patient chooses a mastectomy, she will likely not need radiation therapy unless the tumor is in the axilla (armpit) or invades the chest muscle (pectoralis muscle). The most common complaints with radiation therapy are dry skin, a sunburn effect and fatigue. This is best treated with daily creaming for the skin and rest for the body.

Chemotherapy is given if there is evidence of tumor in the lymph nodes. It is often given to young patients regardless of evidence of spread, although tests based on the physiology of the tumor, such as Mammoprint and Oncotype Dx, are now helping us determine if people need chemotherapy based on the way the tumor behaves.

The Oncotype Dx became incorporated into breast cancer staging in January, 2018. It is performed on 1 cm of tissue after your cancer is removed. The pathology department sends your tumor to a company who examines it for 21 specific genes. It helps decide whether or not your cancer is a type of cancer with a higher risk of returning and whether or not you would benefit from chemotherapy.

The Oncotype test may be sent if you have Stage I, grade 2 or 3 or Stage II, estrogen-receptor positive (ER+), HER-2 and node negative invasive breast cancer. The higher the Oncotype score the more likely a patient may benefit from chemotherapy. A large, therefore powerful, study came out in June 2018 called the TAILORx trial. It found no benefit of chemotherapy in 70% of tumors tested and that for the majority of patients chemotherapy was not more beneficial than surgery, radiation and hormonal therapy.

These patients with tumors that are less than 5 cm, ER+, HER-2 negative, & node-negative where chemotherapy can be avoided are:

* older than 50 with a Oncotype recurrence score of 11-25 (45%)

* any age with a recurrence score of 0-10 (16%)

* 50 years old or younger with a recurrent score of 11-15 (8%)

The findings suggest chemotherapy be considered for the remaining 30% of patients with tumors that are less than 5 cm, ER+, HER-2 negative, & node-negative breast cancer:

* any age with a recurrence score of 26-100 (17%0

* 50 years old or younger with a recurrence score of 16-25 (14%)

Chemotherapy is given in two forms: intravenous (IV) and by mouth (po). IV chemotherapy is given to patients who have evidence of spread of the disease or to those who test at high risk of future metastatic disease. By mouth (po) is given as an antiestrogen agent. Both are prescribed by a medical oncologist and the patient is followed by an oncology team while on any of these medications. Oral chemotherapy medications act to block the growth of tumors by lowering the amount of estrogen that can cause tumor growth. The most common po agents are tamoxifen (Nolvadex), anastrazole (Arimidex), exemestane (Aromasin) and letrozole (Femara).

Most patients who have breast cancer will have a chest x-ray before surgery. Also, blood will be drawn to check blood levels and liver function tests (LFTs) if thought to be indicated. LFTs are checked if there is suspicion the cancer has spread outside the breast. Elevations may be a sign of metastatic disease of the breast to the liver. Bone scans are done if there is suspicion of spread outside the breast, the patient has symptoms of pain, or there is evidence of an increased alkaline phosphatase blood test which may indicate invasion of the bone by cancer. Computerized tomography (CT) scan is performed to check the liver, lungs or brain if indicated.

Surgery will be performed on the breast to remove cancer via mastectomy or partial mastectomy (lumpectomy). Surgery to check lymph nodes in the axilla (armpit) is done for invasive cancer to check for spread outside the breast. Breast cancer has been found to spread from the tumor bed to one or a few lymph nodes before it spreads out to the body (most commonly via the lymphatic and blood streams to the brain, bone, liver and lungs). These guarding or sentinel lymph nodes can be identified and excised for histological analysis. Mapping with Technetium-99m sulfur colloid is done by injecting this radioactive isotope into the areola or tumor area. Using a measuring device, the nodes that are guarding the area are removed surgically. The pathologist then carefully examines these nodes by cutting them like a bread loaf and looking under the microscope for cancer cells within the lymph node. Blue dye (isosulfan blue or methylene blue) is also used to identify sentinel lymph nodes. The major disadvantage of isosulfan blue dye is the risk of life-threatening allergic or anaphylactic reactions leading to hives, low blood pressure, and itching.

In the past, if a sentinel lymph node was found to contain cancer, we would proceed with a full axillary lymph node dissection (ALND), that is, removal of all the lymph nodes in the axilla (armpit). This has a risk of injuring some major nerves (long thoracic and thoracodorsal nerves) and sensory nerves (intercostal nerves) to the upper, inner aspect of the arm. Recent studies such as the Z-0011 trial are supporting the trend to do less and less surgery for breast cancer. The Z-0011 trial states that women with a T1 or T2 Tumor (see Breast Cancer Staging section), no nodal disease, clinically and pathologically proven positive lymph nodes, who are receiving whole breast radiation and an anti-estrogen therapy, have the same recurrence rate and overall survival as those who receive ALND. Therefore, by not performing ALND, women can safely avoid the risks of nerve injury, lymphedema, and motion problems.

Breast cancer is actually many different diseases lumped under one diagnosis. Treatment is individualized based on your type of tumor, your age, Oncotype status and your health. If you are diagnosed, write out your questions in a notebook or on an electronic device to help you remember to ask each and every one. Educate yourself on your tumor type --- its pathology, receptor status, Her-2-neu status, size and possible spread. Ask for the help you need. Most importantly, don't give up hope or faith. Even if you have to face the worst-case scenario, you can expect to live for many more years.

The worst part of breast disease and cancer is the anxiety. Getting help from a therapist, coach or the like is incredibly helpful for all people. The vast majority of people diagnosed with breast cancer do not die from the disease.

Rare types of breast cancer

Two rare forms of breast cancer are Inflammatory Breast Cancer and Paget's Disease of the nipple. With both diseases people often complain of a rash or skin infection of the breast that won't go away even with treatment. With inflammatory breast cancer, you may have dimples, ridges, or redness and warmth on exam. Because this form of breast cancer can spread rapidly, it needs to be diagnosed and treated early and quickly. This is done by sampling of the tissue with biopsy which can often be done via punch biopsy in the office.

It is treated primarily with chemotherapy, but surgery has been found to be helpful in some cases.

Paget's Disease of the nipple begins in the milk ducts and spreads out onto the nipple areolar complex. The skin can appear crusted, red or oozing. Biopsy is the best way to diagnose Paget's Disease. It is treated with surgical excision, radiation and rarely, chemotherapy.

VI. Staging of Breast Cancer

To stage breast cancer, the American Joint Committee on Cancer (AJCC) first places the cancer in a letter category using the TNM classification system. The AJCC is a group of cancer experts who oversee how cancer is classified and communicated. This is to ensure that all doctors and treatment facilities are describing cancer in a uniform way so that the treatment results of all people can be compared and understood.

Traditionally, breast cancer state was calculated using three main factors designated by the letters T, N and M where:

T =tumor size, N=nodal status and M=evidence of metastases.

In 2018, the AJCC updated the breast cancer staging guidelines to add other cancer characteristics to the TNM system to determine breast cancer stage. These include:

  * <u>Tumor grade:</u> a measurement of how much cancer cells look like normal cells. This is on a scale of 1-3. People sometimes confuse this on their pathology report for their stage. Grade is only one component of stage.

* Estrogen and progesterone receptor status (ER & PR):

Do the cancer cells have receptors for the hormones estrogen and progesterone and at what percentage?

* HER-2-neu or HER-2 status: Are the cancer cells making a lot of HER-2 protein?

* Oncotype Dx score: what is the recurrence score (further discussion below)
Once all these factors have been determined, this information is combined in a process called stage grouping to assign an overall stage.

Oncotype Dx Score

In 2018 the use of this well-validated, genomic (looks at the activity of the cancer genes) test was added to the staging of breast cancer. The test is done a block or piece of the cancer tissue removed at the time of surgery. The pathology department sends it to an outside company for testing of 21 genes within the tumor to assess the benefit of chemotherapy in addition to hormonal therapy. It helps predict if your cancer will return and if receiving chemotherapy will decrease the chances of cancer coming back. It is performed on breast cancers that are her-2-neu negative and estrogen receptor (ER) positive. Most insurances cover the cost of the test and it takes about 2-3 weeks for the test to return. This does not delay care as after surgery the next step in therapy (radiation or chemotherapy) does not normally start for one month after surgery is complete.

Soon after surgery, patients' cases are normally presented at Tumor Board where all the practitioners involved in breast care review the medical history, radiology and pathology data and discuss the possibilities of treatment. If your personal medical history and cancer meet criteria for the Oncotype the test is offered to help determine whether or not a patient will benefit from chemotherapy.

The score ranges from 0-100.

Score 0 to 17: Low recurrence score

A low recurrence score is 17 and under.
If you have a low recurrence score, the chance that your cancer will return is low. This also means that the benefits of chemotherapy may not be worth the risks for you. A low recurrence score does not mean that your cancer will definitely not come back.

Score 18 to 30: Medium recurrence score

A medium recurrence score is 18 to 30.
If you have a medium recurrence score, the chance that your cancer will return is in the medium range. The benefits of chemotherapy for you are uncertain. Your doctor will discuss with you what this means.

Score 31 to 100: High recurrence score

A high recurrence score is 31 or over.
If you have a high recurrence score, the chance that your cancer will return is somewhat high. Adding chemotherapy to your cancer treatment may help keep the cancer from coming back.

A high recurrence score does not mean that your cancer will definitely come back.

T: Tumor Size

The letter "T" followed by a number from 0 to 4 describes the tumor size and whether it has spread to the skin or chest wall under the breast. Higher T numbers indicate a larger tumor and/or more extensive spread to the tissues surrounding the breast.

Tx =	Tumor cannot be assessed	
T0 =	No evidence of tumor	
Tis =	LCIS/DCIS/or Paget's Disease not associated with invasive carcinoma	
T1 =	Tumor is 2 cm or less in diameter	
	T1mi =	Tumor $\leq$ 1 mm in greatest dimension
	T1a =	Tumor > 1 mm but $\leq$ 5 mm in greatest dimension
	T1b =	Tumor > 5 mm but $\leq$ 10 mm in greatest dimension
	T1c =	Tumor < 10 mm but $\leq$ 20 mm in greatest dimension
T2 =	Tumor is > than 2 cm to $\leq$ 5 cm in diameter	
T3 =	Tumor is more than 5 cm in diameter	
T4 =	Tumor is any size, has directly extended to the chest wall or is invading through the skin. This includes ulceration, satellite nodules, and edema or the skin	

N: Regional Lymph Nodes

The letter "N" followed by a number from 0 to 3 indicates whether the cancer has spread to the lymph nodes near the breast and, if so, whether the affected nodes are fixed to other structures under the arm. Nodal status is assessed clinically and then again after surgery pathologically. While there are nuances to this I present the clinical assessment here.

Nx =	Regional lymph nodes cannot be assessed (for example, previously removed)	
N0 =	No regional lymph node metastases	
N1 =	Metastases to moveable ipsilateral Level I, II axillary lymph node(s)	
N2 =	Metastases in ipsilateral level I, II axillary lymph nodes that are clinically fixed or matted; or in clinically detected* ipsilateral internal mammary nodes in the absence of clinically evident axillary lymph node metastases	
	N2a =	Metastases in ipsilateral level I, II axillary lymph nodes fixed to one another (matted) or to other structures
	N2b =	Metastases only in clinically detected* ipsilateral internal mammary nodes and in the absence of clinically evident level I, II axillary lymph node metastases
	N3 =	Metastases in ipsilateral infraclavicular (level III axillary) lymph node(s) with or without level I, II axillary lymph node involvement; or in clinically detected* ipsilateral internal mammary lymph node(s) with clinically evident level I, II axillary lymph node metastases; or metastases in ipsilateral supraclavicular lymph node(s) with or without axillary or
	N3a =	Metastases in ipsilateral infraclavicular lymph node(s)
	N3b =	Metastases in ipsilateral internal mammary lymph node(s) and axillary lymph node(s)
	N3c =	Metastases in ipsilateral supraclavicular lymph node(s)

M: Metastasis

The letter "M" followed by a 0 or 1 indicates whether or not the cancer has metastasized (spread) to distant organs (brain, bone, liver, lungs) or to lymph nodes that are not next to the breast, such as those above the collarbone.

Mx =	Metastasis cannot be assessed
M0 =	No clinical or radiographic evidence of distant metastases
M1 =	Distant detectable metastases as determined by classic clinical and radiographic means and/or histologically proven larger than 0.2 mm

TNM Classifications

Outcome if Combine TNM Stage with other High Risk Biomarkers

Stage (7th Edition)	Risk Profile	5-yr. DSS	5-yr. OSS
I	0	100%	97%
(IA abd IB)	1	99.4%	96.7%
	2	98.8%	94.6%
	3	96.6%	93.8%
IIA	0	100%	96.8%
	1	99.4%	97.1%
	2	97.5%	94.1%
	3	91.0%	88.2%
IIB	0	100%	100%
	1	96.9%	94.6%
	2	92.9%	89.3%
	3	91.5%	91.5%
IIIA	0	100%	100%
	1	98.3%	91.5%
	2	92.2%	90.3%
	3	68.6%	68.6%
IIIC	0		
	1	92.2%	84.4%
	2	80.8%	80.8%
	3	33.3%	33.3%

Factor	0 points	1 point
Grade	Grade 1/2	Grade 3
ER status	ER positive	ER Negative
HER2 status	HER2 positive	HER2 negative

Add one point for each of these additional risk factors

DSS = disease specific survival (do not die from breast cancer)
OS = overall survival

Stage 0:	In situ breast cancer, Tis, N0, M0
Stage I:	T1, N0 or N+ only microscopically, M0
Stage IIA:	T0-1, N1, M0 or T2, N0, M0
Stage IIB:	T2, N1, M0 or T3, N0, M0
Stage IIIA:	T0-2, N2, M0 or T3, N1-2, M0
Stage IIIB:	T4, N (any), M0 or T (any), N3, M0
Stave IV:	T (any), N (any), M1

Since January, 2018 we use this former staging model of TNM and use an online calculator including grade, receptor status and Oncotype score (if done) to recalculate your tumor's stage. The biology is now driving treatment which allows for better outcomes and less overtreatment. Adding in these parameters of grade, receptor status and Oncotype score to the TNM staging can upgrade or downgrade your specific stage so ask your doctor to show you the calculation after pathology and testing is complete. Most programs will have a Survivorship meeting at the completion of all treatments (surgery, radiation, chemotherapy and initiation of anti-estrogen therapy). This meeting usually occurs about 9 months after your diagnosis and will assist you in further understanding your cancer and how it has and will change your life. It's hard to believe but many people live more vibrant and fulfilling lives after cancer treatment. And since most people diagnosed with breast cancer today do not die of the disease it often creates positive lifelong changes.

Shared data in 2005 revealed that the overall five-year relative survival rate for female breast cancer patients improved from 63% in the early 1960s to 90% today. This increase is due largely to improvements in treatment (i.e., chemotherapy and hormone therapy) and to widespread use of mammography screening.

The majority of people diagnosed from breast cancer do not die from the disease. Even in Stage IV disease patients can live long and healthy lives with the help of chemotherapeutic agents.

It is a challenging time of emotion and life change. It invokes a grief reaction of mad, sad, bargaining, denial and acceptance. In this stew any of these or other emotions can come up in a nanosecond. It is not a linear or cyclical process. Our goal is to have patients thrive not just survive.

Stage Distribution and 5-year Relative Survival by Stage at Diagnosis of Breast Cancer, All Races, Females

based on the National Cancer Institute SEER data, as of 5/1/2017

		5-year Relative Survival (%)
Stage 0	or Stage 1	close to 100%
Stage 2		93
Stage 3		72
Stage 4		22

One important caveat is that we cannot determine one person's individual outcome or survival.

In summary, the majority of breast cancer is diagnosed at an early stage and therefore, most patients do not die of breast disease. Even the majority of patients with disease that has spread to the lymph nodes live normal lifespans. The good news is that there has been at least a 31% decrease in breast cancer mortality in the last 30 years. With further screening and advances we hope breast cancer deaths will continue to decrease and quality of life to increase.

Surgical Instructions

I. Preoperative instructions   79

II. Postoperative instructions   81

III. Needle Localization   83

IV. Postoperative instructions for life   84

V. Stop, Stay, Sense.....Step (S4r)   86

I. PREOPERATIVE INSTRUCTIONS

Please stop taking aspirin, ibuprofen and Vitamin E at least 10 days prior to surgery. You may take Tylenol. If you take aspirin for your heart, ask the doctor before stopping.

Do not eat or drink after midnight the day before surgery. You may be instructed to take certain medicines with a sip of water the morning of surgery. Please ask if you are not sure. You will be called by the nurses the afternoon prior to surgery with the exact time to arrive.

The risks of surgery of the breast include, but are not limited to: infection, bleeding, need for re-operation, cosmetic deformity, nerve damage and injury to surrounding structures and even death. Other risks relate to you specifically and depend on your medical history. These can include stroke, heart and lung problems, and skin problems.

Expect some bruising after surgery. Ice packs to the area for 15-20 minutes every 2-3 hours can help during the first 24-72 hours after surgery. Buy a bag of peas or two to be used as an ice pack inside a thin towel after surgery.

Call your surgeon if you experience fevers, chills, redness, or have any other problems or questions.

Reddish, pink & yellowish drainage can be normal. Pus (usually white and creamy) is a sign of infection. Call if you notice pus or if you have questions.

The day of surgery you will be checked in and then perhaps need to go to radiology for needle localization and/or lymph node mapping (lymphoscintigraphy). After that you will go the operating room. If you have a biopsy, partial mastectomy, or lymph node surgery you will likely go home the same day of surgery. Full mastectomy (with or without reconstruction) patients may be admitted overnight to the hospital. If so, the majority of patients go home the day after surgery.

II. POSTOPERATIVE INSTRUCTIONS

Dr. Bennett's post-operative instructions for breast surgery

1. Ice pack to the breast or axillary wound in the recovery room and then as much as tolerated over the next 48 hours. At home, you can use two bags of peas. Keep freezing them and wrap one in a kitchen towel. When not cold anymore, switch the bags. Do not eat the peas! This is a great, inexpensive ice pack that won't leak.

2. Walk every day, preferably outside, for at least 15-20 minutes.

3. Rest. Get at least eight hours of sleep each night. You may be tired after surgery and need naps. This may last for up to 6-8 weeks postoperatively. Often the first week is the hardest.

4. Drink fluids. Eat if you want to.

5. Minimize contact with people who are ill.

6. You may shower the day after surgery. Don't rub the incision; pat dry lightly.

7. Remove the dressing if it gets wet or in 48-72 hours. This may happen from a shower (although not usually because the dressing is occlusive) or from drainage from the wound. If the wound drains reddish, yellow or clear fluid, change the dressing and notify your doctor.

8. Call your doctor immediately if you notice signs of infection such as a temperature of 101.5 degrees Fahrenheit or more, pus, redness, warmth, swelling or increasing pain.

9. The wound is weakest at 7-10 days postoperatively. No lifting greater than 10 pounds for one month after surgery. Leave steri-strips in place.

10. Do not drive while taking the narcotic pain medicine. You may drive if you take Tylenol for pain.

11. In brief, your main jobs are to rest, drink water and other healthy fluids, and walk each day.

12. You may wear a bra for comfort. If you are large breasted, you may want to wear a bra for the first week to improve the cosmetic result.

III. NEEDLE LOCALIZATION

A needle or wire localization biopsy is done to mark an area that cannot be felt but it is seen on a radiographic study (mammogram, ultrasound or MRI). A wire is placed at the area of abnormality (and/or prior clip placement) so that the area in question can be sampled or removed. A radiologist and technicians perform the localization procedure.

Before a needle localization of the breast, please do not wear deodorants, powders or perfumes on your upper body.

During the procedure, the technologist will first take preliminary films of the area while you are either lying on a table or in an upright position. While these are reviewed by the radiologist, your breast will remain compressed. Once the area of abnormality is shown on film, the skin is cleansed with a special soap. The radiologist will then anesthetize (numb) your tissues and insert a localizing needle. Films are then taken to show the needles position in relationship to the abnormality. The needle may need to be repositioned. A thin wire is inserted through the needle, and then the needle is withdrawn, leaving the wire in your breast. The wire is bent and taped to your skin. Final films are taken. You may feel the wire in your breast, but generally it is not painful.

After the needle localization has been completed, you will be sent to surgery. The surgeon will use the wire as a guide to find the abnormal area in your breast. A mammogram is done on the tissue removed to make sure the abnormality has been removed. A pathologist then studies the tissue.

IV. POSTOPERATIVE INSTRUCTIONS FOR LIFE

Don't add drama to life (or death). It's actually dramatic enough on its own.

Sleep when you can. Eat when you can.

Don't poke a skunk.

Prepare and get everything you need before the procedure.

Postoperative instructions for self-care and life: Rest. Walk every day. Drink water. Take care of your body. When you are tired or recuperating that is enough.

Listen to your body.

Occam's razor: there is likely one reason to explain an outcome.

Being tired is not an excuse for being mean. Or anything else.

Focus. See the big picture and the small. Widen your lens to see the earth, the forest and the trees. Make it small too to see the leaves, the details, the roots.

Don't make good perfect. That's when complications occur.

Good enough is perfect.

Slow down. Take time to play which is defined as time spent without purpose.

Always do your best. And then accept good enough. Perfection is the enemy of good.

Beware the voice of experience. Why?

Where does good judgment come from? Experience.

Where does experience come from?

Bad judgment.

Mistakes are the best teachers in life. Try not to make mistakes that kill people. Celebrate all other mistakes and learn from them.

Always do your best. Always. Even if you have to dig deeper within yourself than you believe you can. Because there is actually more there. You can do so much more than you think you can. Trust your body. It can keep going.

The body doesn't lie. Trust it.

Parents who are connected to their children know more than any study or test. Listen to them.

Cultivate calm and stillness. Breathing helps cultivate calm and stillness.

Always tell the truth.

If you don't know, say, "I don't know." Knowing your limits and telling what you don't know saves lives.

Multitasking is not possible. What we call multitasking is being able to quickly and smoothly change our focus from one task to the next. I imagine it like changing from one thing to the next without any tendrils connecting me to the first task. Strive for complete attention to each thing you are doing or person you are with.

Cultivate laughter, song and dance.

V. STOP, STAY, SENSE.....STEP

Stop, Stay, Sense, Step.....Repeat (S4r)

I see this pattern repeated over and over again in a variety of secular and non-secular teachings. I offer it here to you. It can help you get present to what is.

<u>Stop:</u> Stop. Sacred Pause.

We must pause for a Time Out before we begin surgery when we check the patient's information and surgery we are planning on performing. Pausing and checking in lessens mistakes in the operating room and can have a profound positive effect on our lives as well.

I often imagine putting my hand out with the palm flat or put my hand to my heart to offer a bit of self-compassion. Stop moving, stop doing, and detach from your thoughts. It may help to remember that you are not your thoughts or feelings. Your mind may continue on. Taking a breath can help our bodies stop and decrease our heart and breathing rates as well as sweating. Deep breaths activate nerves that calm our bodies and minds.

<u>Stay:</u> Begin to feel into the moment. Even if flight/fight/freeze has kicked in, please stay for a moment. Stay with the pause, the breath, or even a sensation within your body. It can help to realize in this moment you are safe.

<u>Sense:</u> Tune into your senses. Begin to observe. Begin to name. What do you smell? See? Hear? Taste? Feel on your skin?

Notice within your body? Once, an eighth grade student noticed that we even may have a sense beyond our typical 5 senses.....can you notice if that is true for you? It may be the most important sense we have.

In the step of Sense pay attention to what is. Within you and around you. Notice, name and observe. It can help to begin by feeling your hands and feet. The feet and hands can be an entry point into noticing what is happening within the body. It is also helpful to tune into where you are to separate a bit from thoughts.

Trust your body. It does not lie. The problem is that we can notice what is happening within our bodies but often our imagination and stories cultivate fear, not calm, truth or love. We have 10x more neurons in our gut/gastrointestinal system than we do in our brain. That gut instinct we speak of is critical. Learning to live from our gut and heart over our head helps us live happier, healthier lives.

<u>Step:</u> What is your next step? Is it a physical step? A letting go? Notice up to three next steps (no more than three) from this moment for you.

<u>Repeat:</u> Repeat over and over. The path is forgetting and remembering and stopping, staying and sensing will help you keep stepping through your life.

VII. Additional Resources

Websites:

www.drkerrybennett.com

www.breastcancer.org

www.cancer.org

www.komen.org

www.amazon.com and other bookstores have a wide variety of books available.

A word to the wise regarding research on the internet and the impact of sharing your story with others. Our society catastrophizes and dramatizes. For some reason, when people find out they have breast cancer, they are often faced with people around them telling them the horror stories they have heard or witnessed. Instead of listening, they offer stories, for some reason worst case scenario stories. Be careful. I tell each of my patients to pretend they have a button the can press to put SHIELDS UP! Newly diagnosed patients need to protect themselves from the well-meaning stories of others while they struggle to learn about their particular tumor and its characteristics. The internet is full of "false news" that cultivates fear, promotes products and prays on people who are trying to take good care of themselves. People who are happy and living their lives often do not post on the internet so there is selection bias on the net. Just ask! We are here to support you and answer all of your questions.

There may be thousands of different breast cancers. Each cancer is unique as is each individual. We are learning more about how these tumors behave and finding ways to differentiate them. At this point, breast cancer treatment is based primarily on pathology, but as we learn more about the biology and genetics of tumors this will change treatment patterns.

If you have breast cancer it is your mountain to get over and you need help and support. Find doctors and caretakers with whom you feel comfortable being yourself and who will give you the information you need to make your individual choices.

Transforming Fear

Fear keeps us stuck. Fear-based decisions almost always backfire. Therefore, I have found that one of the main focuses of my work as an oncology surgeon is to help decrease and eliminate fear. I hope to create safety and trust and empower my patients to co-create decisions for their best health.

Dick Schwartz, Ph.D. who founded Internal Family Systems (IFS) states a law of inner physics is "there is nothing inside you that can hurt you or has any power if you are not afraid it —- if you are in Self." He characterizes Self as containing the qualities of clarity, calm, compassion, courage, confidence, connection, creativity and curiosity as well as patience, persistence, playfulness, presence and perspective.

In cancer basing choices on truth and not the "false news" present on the internet or by well-meaning but fear-based stories of friends. The anticipation is taking the steps needed such as good self-care, surgery, radiation or medicines as well as having support of friends, family, a therapist, nutritionist, physical therapist and other caregivers.

In our fear-based society there is so much misinformation about cancer. For example: Do you think the majority of people who express breast cancer have a family history? Based on the current media one would naturally think that answer is definitely yes. But the truth is 85% of people who get breast cancer do not have a family history. Get the facts and truth and that will help you move from fear to true, not false, hope.

The truth really does set us free.

A poem prayer

by Kerry

Release the past and it's pain

Release the future and it's fear

Embrace the lessons of the past

Embrace the joy, hope and trust of the future

Live and love in the present

Create from there

Thank you